The Treatment of Horses
by
Homœopathy

by

G. MacLeod
M.R.C.V.S., D.V.S.M.
ASSOCIATE OF THE FACULTY OF HOMOEOPATHY

VETERINARY CONSULTANT TO MESSRS A. NELSON & CO
HOMOEOPATHIC PHARMACY, LONDON

VETERINARY CONSULTANT TO THE BRITISH
HOMOEOPATHIC ASSOCIATION

Index by Maurice Prior

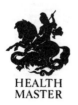

HEALTH
MASTER

HEALTH SCIENCE PRESS,
HENGISCOTE, BRADFORD,
HOLSWORTHY, DEVON.

ISBN 0 85032155 7

Printed in Great Britain by
Clarke Doble & Brendon Ltd., Plymouth, Devon.

CONTENTS

INTRODUCTION

Colleagues have sometimes asked for the literature on which veterinary homoeopathic medicine is based. My earlier replies were that a study of the principles of Homoeopathy is necessary before attempting its application to veterinary work, for that had been my own approach. In recent years, it has been found more helpful to involve a colleague in the treatment of a dog, cat, herd of cattle or promising race-horse before recommending literature. The independent judgment of such a colleague is of the greatest value, evidenced by an increasing desire to study the subject. It is doubtful, however, if this work on horses would have been undertaken had there not been frequent requests from horse-owners for a text-book on horses which might clarify their own approach to Homoeopathy. There are many knowledgeable homoeopaths in this country, whose private study is admirable, but among them has been an increasing awareness of the need to relate knowledge of the subject to a better understanding of the remedies which may be used.

It is clear that degrees of knowledge vary so much that it is advisable to stress the main differences between the traditional and the homoeopathic assessment of an animal's health. In the loss of health, whatever the cause, the conventional approach has been to have the condition diagnosed and it is this which is regarded as of first importance in the treatment. The homoeopath accepts the diagnosis and then extends his observation of the animal to note all the evidence of loss of health and use such evidence to select appropriate treatment to restore the animal to good health. This approach for the beginner is not easy and even after considerable successes in the selection of suitable remedies, it should never be thought easy.

Case-histories have been examined and arranged in a manner which could be related to horse affections in standard text-books. The homoeopathic materia medica is vast, so it should be remembered that the remedies listed are by no means the only ones which may be applicable. They are remedies which have been used and, in several cases, very well tried. A few diseases not encountered, either because they are uncommon in Britain, or occur only in other countries, have been included and the remedies listed for these conditions are but suggested courses of treatment.

I acknowledge, with gratitude, the constant encouragement of the Faculty of Homoeopathy, the British Homoeopathic Association and Mr. J.B.L. Ainsworth of Nelson's Pharmacy, London.

G. Macleod, M.R.C.V.S., D.V.S.M.

THE HOMOEOPATHIC APPROACH

As in all homoeopathic medicine, whether human or veterinary, treatment is based on the totality of symptoms presented and not on the condition which has been diagnosed. This does not mean that the diagnosis is unimportant. The homoeopath accepts the diagnosis, but extends his observation of the patient to note individual symptoms which may not be thought, by orthodox standards, to have any significance. If all the animal's symptoms can be studied, the appropriate remedy may be found. The facts referred to as symptoms include the animal's individual characteristics, its preferences, its sudden departure from normal behaviour. In addition to symptoms, the animal's previous medical history is also important. It follows, therefore, that in the application of homoeopathy to veterinary medicine, the owner of the animal should be acutely observant. The veterinary surgeon who is a homoeopath may notice symptoms which the owner has missed, because the animal's behaviour is familiar and not thought to be important. The combined observations will assist the selection of the remedy.

Before further explanation of the approach to homoeopathic medicine, it should be stressed that it is not intended as a substitute for surgical intervention where surgery is indicated. There exists a common misconception that doctors and veterinary surgeons who are homoeopaths will avoid operations where these are necessary and thereby submit the patient to "useless" medication. The use of correct homoeopathic treatment has undoubtedly saved animals from *unnecessary* surgery provided treatment has begun before there has been lengthy neglect, resulting in significant destruction of tissue. A few examples of medical treatment given immediately the patient's pain was noticed by the owner can be found under Poll evil and Fistulous Withers.

The homoeopathic approach is often hard to accept, for the

Materia Medica offers no easy short, or even long, list of specific remedies for any disease. The orthodox materia medica concerns itself mainly with substantial dosage of medicines and studies the action of these medicines on the system. Homoeopathy is concerned with materia medica in the fullest sense of the term, with discovery and preparation of medicinal substances and their testing, expressing dosage of a medicine in minute amounts, sufficient to bring about vital stimulation of the cell and leading to a vital reaction of the affected tissue. Symptoms are indicative of a disturbance of the vital process within the animal and should be regarded as evidence that the system is reacting to the stimulus of a disease-producing agent and is endeavouring to overcome the undesirable effects of that agent. Homoeopathic remedies, instead of suppressing these symptoms, aid the healing process by vital stimulation of the body's defences by natural means.

The most simple way to illustrate the importance of individual symptoms is to consider, at this point, one condition. The tried remedies for cases of Epistaxis are twelve in number, see section V. There is a brief record of horses suffering from nose-bleed, but all of them showing slightly different symptoms, so different remedies were used. In some cases, it had been accepted that, prior to homoeopathic treatment, the condition would recur. After homoeopathic treatment, recurrence was found to be rare and a frequent comment from the owner expressed surprise that other symptoms, not thought to be important enough to report, had disappeared and the horse seemed to be in much better general health. This last comment becomes more frequent the more one pursues the satisfying study of homoeopathic medicine.

Having selected the remedy, potencies and frequency of dosage require equal care. It is seldom advisable to make general statements about the use of potencies, for experience shows that there are exceptions to the use of low potencies for chronic ill-health and the higher potencies for acute illness. In cases recorded, chronic conditions needed treatment over a long period, from ten days to a month or longer, with infrequent dosage, while acute cases needed more frequent dosage over a much shorter period. The use of very high potencies is not advisable, except under professional supervision, since it is essential that the severity of the condition is understood and related to the function of the remedy in its chosen potency. Frequency of dosage and duration of treatment are often mistakenly overdone by beginners, mainly because they are mindful of the infinitesimal dose but not appreciating the stimulus of potentised medicine. If due care is given to frequency of dosage and length of treatment, it is advisable to cease treatment when improvement has been noted.

HOMOEOPATHIC MATERIA MEDICA

Although there is an abundance of valuable literature already available on the principles governing Homoeopathy, the works on materia medica are based on the subjective symptoms of human beings. A veterinary materia medica, for obvious reasons, would be based entirely on objectivity. Several horse-breeders who are homoeopaths have asked for a materia medica which would assist their study and appreciation of the subject. It may be sufficient to outline a few of the commoner remedies so frequently recurring in many following chapters.

ACONITUM NAPELLUS (Monk's Hood or Wolf's Bane), a member of the natural order Ranunculaceae, is extremely poisonous. In the preparation of the mother tincture, the entire plant is used as all parts contain the active principle, an alkaloid — Aconitine. The plant has an affinity with serous membranes and muscular tissues leading to functional disturbances. *Aconitum* is the first remedy to be considered in all fevers and inflammatory states. It is especially indicated in complaints which have their origin in exposure to cold dry winds and also in conditions associated with severe fright. Shivering, with cold sweats, usher in the illness which calls for *Aconitum.* Severe respiratory distress may be evident. The upper parts of the body may be hot, in contrast to the colder lower areas. The expression of the animal indicates a state of acute anxiety and there is thirst for large quantities of cold water.

BELLADONNA (The Deadly Nightshade) belongs to the natural order Solanaceae. The berries are extremely poisonous. *Belladonna* produces its action on every part of the nervous system, resulting in a state of excitement and active congestion

There is a marked action on the vascular system, skin and glands. The horse which requires *Belladonna* exhibits characteristic symptoms of dilated pupils, full bounding pulse and a burning hot skin. There are frequent muscular twitchings or jerkings and possibly convulsions. Aggressive tendencies may become exaggerated and the horse may bite and kick at any object. Conditions which call for this remedy are worsened by noise, bright light or any jarring or jerking. During treatment with *Belladonna*, the horse should be confined to a quiet, warm loose-box.

CALCAREA FLUORICA (Fluorspar is the origin) crystals are found in the bone canals. This increases the hardness and, in excess, produces a brittleness. It also occurs in tooth enamel and the epidermis. Affinity with the above-mentioned tissues suggests a liability to form exostoses and enlargement of glands. There is also involvement of veins. The special sphere of this remedy in relation to bone and glandular structures makes it a valuable one for exosteses of bones and indurations of glands.

RHUS TOXICODENDRON is commonly known as Poison Ivy. The mother tincture is prepared from the freshly gathered leaves just before flowering. The plant produces an itchy skin within forty-eight hours of contact, leading to papule formation followed by vesicles which may last up to one week. The vesicular eruption may spread to mucous membranes. Muscular weakness is prominent and there may be an associated muscular stress, producing sprains and strains. One of the main characteristics of the remedy and a main guide to its use is that conditions improve from movement and worsen at rest. It is frequently called for in the many lamenesses which may result from incidents during exercise.

ARSENICUM ALBUM, prepared from Arsenic trioxide, acts on every tissue of the body and its characteristic symptoms provide a most useful guide to its selection. Restlessness is a key sign, the horse invariably changing position frequently. Thirst for small quantities occurs and symptoms are made worse towards, or after, midnight. Discharges are usually acrid and burning tending to excoriate the skin. The skin is markedly affected and the remedy frequently called for in the many conditions which affect it, a guiding symptom being dryness accompanied by scurf and attended by pruritus. It is also of great value in respiratory conditions, post-influenzal weakness responding well to the remedy in the form of its iodide – *Arsenicum Iodatum.*

HEPAR SULPHURIS CALCAREUM is a form of Calcium sulphide. Conditions are characterised by extreme sensitivity, e.g. to pain in the nervous system. The mucous membranes of the alimentary and respiratory tracts are also susceptible to its influence, characterised here by a catarrhal inflammation and tendency to pus formation: This suppurative tendency extends also to the skin and lymphatic system. Thirst may be excessive. There is great liability to sepsis, any small injury leading to infection. In the early stage of inflammation, this remedy in high potency, e.g. 200c – 1M may abort the process, while lower potencies, e.g. 6x – 6c may hasten discharge of purulent material.

HYPERICUM PERFORATUM (St. John's Wort) is the source of a great nerve remedy. The mother tincture is prepared from the whole plant. The red colour of the juice from the expressed plant contains Hypericin, a glucoside which may cause photo-sensitisation in skewbald or piebald animals. This in turn can result in liver dysfunction leading to jaundice, along with sloughing and necrosis of non-pigmented areas. The main affinity of the plant is with the nervous system, causing hyper-sensitivity. There is excessive tenderness of affected parts. Jerking and twitching of muscles occur. A prominent symptom is extreme sensitivity to pain or touch over the region of the lower spine. This remedy is of the greatest value in lacerated wounds involving nerves and is an important adjunct in the treatment of tetanus. The animal is worse from exposure to cold and better at rest.

APIS MELLIFICA is prepared from the entire honey-bee. Bee venom possesses haemolytic, haemorrhagic and neurotoxic effects in addition to its histamine activity. Oedema leading to effusion is the central effect of the action of the remedy *Apis.* The venom produces local and systemic symptoms, the former appearing as swelling containing fluid, the latter as various degrees of urticaria and oedema which may affect any organ. Symptoms of illness may be acute and violent, leading to widespread swellings. Serous effusions occur into body cavities. This is a remedy for which there are many uses in work with horses, for it is indicated in any condition where oedema and serous effusion occur. It usually promotes urination.

NUX VOMICA or poison nut belongs to the natural order Loganiaceae. The dried seeds of the plant are used in the preparation of the mother tincture and contain the alkaloids strychnine and brucine. The alkaloid strychnine has a tissue affinity for the nervous system, especially the motor elements of the spinal cord. The horse which needs *Nux vom.* as a remedy has a poor appetite with attendant constipation. Digestive upsets brought on by unsuitable food will benefit from its use. There may also be muscular twitchings.

BRYONIA (Wild Hops) is a hedgerow plant, the root stock of which is used in the manufacture of the mother tincture. The plant contains a glucoside which is capable of producing severe purgation. *Bryonia* exerts its action on epithelial tissues, serous and synovial membranes and some mucous surfaces producing an inflammatory response resulting in a fibrinous or serous exudate. This in turn leads to dryness of affected parts and effusions into synovial cavities. Movement of parts is interfered with and this produces one of the main indications for its use, viz. all symptoms are worse on movement. Illness which calls for this remedy is slow to develop, in contrast to *Aconitum* or *Belladonna*. The horse prefers to lie still, as movement increases its discomfort. Firm pressure on an affected area relieves the condition, e.g. over the ribs in pleurisy. This explains the preference of the animal to lie on the affected side. The condition is also aggravated by heat, and also in the late evening and early morning. Cold applications provide relief.

ARNICA is a member of the natural order Compositae and is known in its natural habitat as "Fall Herb". The mother tincture is prepared from the root, flowers and leaves. The action of this plant on the system is practically synonymous with a state resulting from injuries or blows, being used primarily for wounds and injuries where the skin remains unbroken, as in bruising. It has a marked affinity with blood-vessels leading to dilation and stasis, with increased permeability. Various types of haemorrhage can thus occur. It also produces diarrhoea tremors and convulsions. Its affinity with muscle can lead to hypertrophy, e.g. enlarged heart. There are skin rashes and eruptions which may be vesicular in type. This is a main remedy to combat shock and should be given as a routine measure before and after operations and also after parturition.

Further information is available elsewhere in homoeopathic literature. In addition to the remedies listed in Part II, there is mention of nosodes. These are disease products, obtained from any affected part of the system and thereafter potentised, e.g. *Influenzinum*, made from the respiratory secretion of affected animals. In specific, i.e. bacterial, viral or protozoal disease, the causative organism may, or may not, be present in the material and the efficacy of the nosode in no way depends on the organism being present. The response of the tissue to invasion by bacteria or viruses results in the formation of substances which are in effect the basis of the nosode.

An oral vaccine is prepared from the actual organism which causes disease and may derive from filtrates containing only the exotoxins of the bacteria, or from emulsions containing both bacteria and their toxins. These filtrates and emulsions are then potentised and become oral vaccines. The two terms "nosode" and "homoeopathic oral vaccine" have come to be regarded as synonymous. They are used both as preventive measures and in treatment.

PREPARATION OF HOMOEOPATHIC REMEDIES

Homoeopathic preparations may be described as medicaments produced from material described in homoeopathic MATERIA MEDICA or PHARMACOPOEIA, by particular methods enabling them to be used in homoeopathic treatment. The Hahnemann process of serial dilution with succussion is considered advisable when medicines in dilution are to be produced for employment in homoeopathic treatment. The preparations customarily are described by the use of the old latin name of the drug, substance or composition employed, followed by the conventional designation of the dilution, the following symbols being used:

> Ø for mother tinctures — the concentrated form of the medicament,
>
> x or D (Continental) for decimal dilution,
>
> c or cH (Continental) for centesimal dilution,

preceded or followed by a number expressing the degree of dilution. Tablets, pills, trituration, granules, powder doses and liquid preparations all take the denomination of the dilution used.

The starting material for the dilutions prepared according to the Hahnemann method may be mother tinctures, chemical products of natural or synthetic origin, biological preparations in the widest sense and any substance which may be considered of medicinal value. Many of the basic materials used in the preparation of homoeopathic medicines do not appear in standard pharmaceutical reference books.

The nomenclature used in homoeopathy has remained virtually unchanged from its introduction in the early part of the 19th century to the present day.

There are two methods of designating the degree of dilution present in the medication, that based on dilution in 10's and that based on dilution in 100's. The 10's scale is termed the decimal and the 100's scale, centesimal.

In the U.K. relatively few strengths are denoted as decimal, but the following will be seen particularly in the older textbooks:

$$1x = 1/10 = 10^{-1}$$
$$3x = 1/1000 = 10^{-3}$$
$$6x = 1/1000000 = 10^{-6}$$
$$12x = 1/1000000000000 = 10^{-12}$$

The centesimal scale is much more frequently used, and the following numerals will be seen in the literature:

> 3 which is a dilution of $1/1000000 = 10^{-6}$
>
> 6 which is a dilution of $1/1000000000000 = 10^{-12}$
>
> 12 which is a dilution of 10^{-24}
>
> 30 which is a dilution of 10^{-60}
>
> 200 which is a dilution of 10^{-400}
>
> 1000
>
> Or 1M which is a dilution of 10^{-2000}

The numbers are the conventional signs of homoeopathic medicine used to denote the strength or potency of preparation required. The strength denotes the degree of dilution of the solution used to moisten the solid forms of medicaments: tablets, pills or powder, etc.

The method of achieving the dilutions in the pharmacy is by use of individual containers which are filled to a predetermined capacity to provide a means of serial dilution, usually by 1 part in 100 parts in successive stages, thus it is necessary to utilise 6 vials to produce the 6c (10^{-12}) potency,

12 vials for the   12 (10^{-24})
30 vials for the   30 (10^{-60})
200 vials for the 200 (10^{-400}) and so on. At each separate stage of dilution the mixture is vigorously shaken, a process termed succussion.

It is apparent that the commonly used potencies of 6, 12, 30, 200 etc. do not contain any material quantity of the original solution in any preparation and it is evidently some intangible energy which is being produced and transferred to the solid dispensing forms. Consequently it is possible to produce tablets, etc. by addition of drops of the required potency in redistilled ethanol.

The form of the medicament considered most practical for administering doses to animals is the sugar granule unit dose.

These are available in individual glass tubes each containing about 1 gramme of preparation.

Where it is necessary to administer doses in the drinking water liquid forms also are prepared.

I General Pathological Conditions

1. Inflammation. This is the process by which nature brings about healing of any damaged part, and can result from mechanical or bacterial cause, the latter being the more serious.

SYMPTOMS
There are four cardinal signs generally described as heat, swelling, redness and pain. The third, of course, is seldom recognisable in the horse. Swelling varies according to the location of the inflammation, e.g. it is more obvious in tissues which are plentifully supplied with blood. Pain is dependent on the amount of damage to nerve endings. A chronic form of inflammation can arise as a result of repeated irritation of a part and in this case the four signs mentioned above will be absent. Chronic inflammation leads to the formation of fibrous tissue during the healing process. The inflammatory process may resolve under treatment, but if neglected can lead to septic involvement or possibly death of tissue.

TREATMENT
Aconitum napellus 6c   In all cases, give early. Dose: two hourly for four doses.
Belladonna 1M   Pronounced heat, with smooth skin, possibly dilated pupils and full pulse. Dose: two hourly for four doses.
Ferrum phosphoricum 6x   Local inflammation of vascular parts leading to congestion. Dose: three hourly for three doses.
Cantharis 6c   Blistery or vesicular inflammation where the guiding symptom is excessive pain and burning heat, sometimes associated with strangury. Dose: two hourly for four doses.
Rhus toxicodendron 1M   Vesicular type inflammatory rash leading to severe pruritis. Dose: once daily for seven days.
Arnica 30c   Superficial inflammation resulting from injury.

Dose: two doses two hours apart.

Silicea 200c   In chronic inflammation, this remedy will help reabsorb fibrous tissue. Dose: once daily for seven days.

Hepar sulphuris 200c   In neglected cases, suppuration may occur. Dose: night and morning for four days.

Note: —   Specific inflammations are considered in their appropriate chapters.

2.   **Abscesses.**   An abscess arises when the skin is broken, allowing entrance to the wound of pyogenic bacteria. Abscesses also occur as a result of generalised pyaemic states. They may be either hot (acute) or cold, and yield pus of varying character according to the type of infection. In slow forming abscesses it is not uncommon for the pus to become insipissated when it appears as a cheese-like mass.

SYMPTOMS

Accute inflammation accompanies the formation of a superficial abscess and appears as a rounded firm swelling which becomes more tense as the condition progresses and the abscess matures. Systemic symptoms are uncommon in this type. Deep abscesses involve subcutaneous and deeper tissues and may be accompanied by febrile disturbances such as rapid pulse and shallow respiration. This type of abscess occurs in the course of pyogenic infections such as joint-ill, brucellosis, etc.

TREATMENT

Hepar sulphuris 30c   Acute abscesses, when area is sensitive to touch and pain severe. Dose: two hourly for four doses.

Mercurius corrosivus 200c   Abscess yields greenish pus streaked with blood. Necrotic ulcers remaining after abscess has ruptured. Dose: three times daily for two days.

Kali Bichromicum 30c   Yellowish stringy pus, difficult to expel. Dose: three times daily for three days.

Silicea 200c   Chronic or cold abscess, pus thin and creamy. Dose: once daily for seven days.

Sulphur iodatum 6c   Multiple small abscesses in various parts. Dose: night and morning for five days.

Anthracinum 30c   Abscess surrounded by hard ring and bluish-black discolouration of the adjacent skin. Dose: once daily for four days.

Tarentula cubensis 30c   General septic state leading to burning abscesses with a purplish colour, with threatened death of tissue. Dose: two hourly for four doses.

Externally, once the abscess has opened, an application once or twice daily of combined *Calendula* and *Hypericum* lotion will assist healing.

Note: —   Nosodes such as *Streptococcus, Staphylococcus* and *Brucella abortus* will be useful, subject to the identification of the organism concerned.

3.   **Ulcers.**   The term ulcer implies a wound which involves any destruction of tissue, superficial or deep, and shows little tendency to heal. Ulceration may arise as a result of the presence in the wound of dead tissue resulting from deprivation of nerve supply. Weakness of blood supply may also contribute to the formation of an ulcer, which may be seen in the course of many specific diseases.

SYMPTOMS

The ulcer usually takes the form of a rounded area, either superficial or deep and may be raised above the level of the surrounding skin or level with it. There is usually an accompanying discharge which is at first serous but soon becomes purulent as a result of secondary infection.

TREATMENT

Mercurius sol. 30c   Main ulcer is surrounded by small pimples. Ulcer yields a blood-streaked greenish pus and is usually irregular in shape rather than rounded. Dose: three times daily for four days.

Calcarea sulphurica 6c   Ulcer has yellowish crust, discharging creamy pus. Dose: three times daily for four days.

Anthracinum 30c   Severe burning heat round ulcer. Skin blackish and hard. Discharge of foul material. Dose: once daily for four days.

Echinacea 3x   Tends to return after healing. Associated lymphatic glands enlarged. Dose: three times daily for three days.

Fluoric acid 6c   Ulcers with red edges surrounded by vesicles. Pruritis is common. Strong-smelling perspiration. Dose: three times daily for four days.

Lachesis 30c   Ulcers associated with a purplish or bluish discolouration of skin. Ulceration round veins. Dose: three hourly for four doses.

Nitric acid 200c   Superficial ulcers which bleed easily. Sensitive and have indefinite edges. Dose: once daily for one week.

Hepar sulphuris 200c   Excessive sensitivity to touch. Foul-smelling pus and in acute cases may contain blood. Older ulcers slow to heal and are accompanied by severe pruritis. Dose: two hourly for four doses.

Silicea 200c   Chronic ulcer showing tendency to burrow deeply and form fistulae. Dose: once daily for seven days.

Externally, a lotion of Calendula will aid materially in the healing process.

4.   Sinus and Fistula.   The term sinus implies an indolent tract of tissue which discharges purulent material. Fistula implies a tract which opens on the surface of the skin from a deeper tissue. The two names, however, have become almost synonymous. A sinus or blind fistula arises as a result of a deep wound or abscess discharging its material on the surface of the skin. Necrotic tissue deep in the wound can contribute to it, along with poor drainage from the deeper tissues. Sinuses and fistulae may be associated with specific conditions such as Poll Evil, Fistulous Withers and other diseases.

SYMPTOMS

The opening of the fistula or sinus varies in size and the surrounding tissues may show granulations or fibrosis according to the age of the lesion. Secondary fistulae may appear and connect with the main one. The purulent discharge may heal and then break out again once new deep-seated abscesses mature. The pus which is discharged may be blood-stained and is invariably foul-smelling.

TREATMENT

Hepar sulphuris 200c   Inflammatory symptoms accompany sinus. Tissues extremely sensitive to touch. Dose: two hourly for four doses.

Mercurius sol. 30c   Sinus discharges greenish thin pus streaked with blood. Surrounding tissues show small pimples or vesicles. Dose: three times daily for three days.

Kali bichromicum 30c   Pus is tough and stringy, yellow, expressed with difficulty. Dose: three times daily for four days.

Silicea 200c   Chronic involvement, pus thin and greyish, fibrous tissue forming. Dose: once daily for seven days. Useful in recurrent outbreaks. Dose: night and morning for seven days.

Calcarea fluorica 30c   Sinus opening surrounded by hard elevated edges, with swelling of skin. Pus is thick and yellow. Dose: night and morning for seven days.

Externally the sinus tract should be irrigated with a solution of *Calendula* and *Hypericum.*

5.   **Wounds.**   Wounds may be open or external, or closed or internal. Open wounds are usually due to some form of external damage and take the form of incised, contused, lacerated or punctured.

SYMPTOMS

Primary signs include pain and possible haemorrhage, while secondary involvement shows in the form of repair, which may take various forms, including suppuration. There may be febrile involvement if the wound is extensive or is deep and punctured.

TREATMENT

Arnica 30c   Give always as a routine remedy, especially in contused wounds. Dose: Two doses two hours apart.

Hypericum 1M   Lacerated wounds where nerve endings have been damaged and pain is obvious. Dose: two hourly for four doses.

Ledum 6c   Deep punctured wounds. Surrounding skin cold and bluish. Dose: two hourly for four doses.

Calendula 6c   This remedy will assist healing of tissues. Dose: three times daily for one day.

Externally a lotion made up of equal parts of *Calendula*, and *Hypericum* will be of great assistance in promoting healing.

Note: —   The combination of *Ledum* and *Hypericum* internally will be helpful in the prevention of tetanus and should always be given when a wound is likely to become infected.

6.   **Burns and Scalds.**   Various lesions result from burns, depending on the area of the skin involved and the depth of

penetration. Burns which affect a large area are more serious than smaller deep burns.

TREATMENT

Aconitum napellus 6c   The use of this remedy will obviate the effects of shock and will allay fear. Dose: every two hours for four doses.

Arnica 30c   A useful routine remedy which should be given as soon as possible. Dose: two doses two hours apart.

Cantharis 6c   Blisters, severe pain, skin hot and swollen. Dose: two hourly for four doses.

Urtica urens 6c   Mild burns showing watery blisters with tendency to itch. Dose: three hourly for four doses.

Apis 6c   Oedema of subcutaneous tissues remaining after initial symptoms have subsided. Dose: two hourly for four doses.

Externally the application of a burn ointment containing *Cantharis, Urtica urens* and *Apis* will be most helpful. A compress of *Calendula* lotion will also be of considerable value.

II Affections of the Eye

1. Contusion of the Eyeball.   This may arise from any blow inflicted by a blunt object.

SYMPTOMS
Small purpura-like haemorrhages are seen underneath the conjunctiva. Larger extravasations of blood accumulate in the anterior chamber of the eye. Severe injury may result in rupture of the sclera or cornea.

TREATMENT
Arnica 30c   This should be given as soon as possible after
   occurrence of the injury. Dose: two doses three hours apart.
Hypericum 1M   Intense pain associated with injury to nerves
   and soft structures. Dose: three times daily for two days.
Externally a lotion made up of *Calendula*, and *Hypericum* will be of benefit, aiding the action of internal remedies. The dilution should be one in ten, and applied two or three times daily until improvements set in.

2. Open Wounds of the Eyeball.   Such wounds, caused by any sharp pointed instrument may be either penetrating or non-penetrating. The former involve the iris and other surfaces as deep as the retina, while the latter involve the outer parts such as cornea and conjunctiva.

TREATMENT
A lotion made of *Calendula, Arnica* and *Hypericum* should be used to irrigate the eye two or three times daily. Use ten drops to a half-pint of warm water. Internally, the following remedies should be considered:-
Arnica 30c   This remedy should always be given in an injury to
   combat shock and hasten recovery. Dose: one dose three

hourly for two doses should suffice.

Hypericum 1M   Pain caused by laceration of and injury to nerves and also helps to control haemorrhage. Dose: one dose two hourly for four doses.

Ledum 6c   Penetrating, deep wounds. It can profitably be combined with Hypericum to relieve pain and prevent complications. Dose: one dose two hourly for four doses.

Hepar sulphuris 6c   In this low potency, the remedy will help promote healing and discharge of pus, if secondary infection leads to purulent involvement. Dose: one dose three hourly for four doses.

3. Conjunctivitis.   This term implies inflammation of the conjunctiva, the membrane covering the eye or the under-surface of the eyelid. It may arise from injuries or irritation from some extraneous matter.

SYMPTOMS

The eyelids become swollen and lachrymation occurs. Photophobia is intense and the eyelids remain closed in severe cases. Dullness of the cornea is evident. Acute cases are accompanied by febrile symptoms such as rapid pulse and respiration. Mucopurulent material gathers in the corners of the eye as the condition progresses. The cornea shows increased vascularity.

TREATMENT

Aconitum napellus 6c   Early stages showing febrile symptoms. Dose: every hour for four doses.

Belladonna 1M   Animal excitable showing rapid pulse and dilated pupils. The skin is hot and shiny, patchy sweating occurs. Dose: two hourly for four doses.

Euphrasia 6c   Profuse lachrymation and photophobia. Dose: three times daily for two days.

Mercurius sol 30c   Discharge becomes purulent and has greenish tinge. Salivation and slimy diarrhoea may be present. Dose: three times daily for two days.

Nux vomica 6c   Digestive upsets accompany condition. Dose: three times daily for two days.

Arnica 30c   When condition has its origin in any form of injury. Dose: two doses, three hours apart.

Hypericum 1M   Signs of intense pain. Conjunctival blood-vessels become congested and prominent. Dose: two hourly for four doses.

Externally, a lotion of *Hypericum* and *Calendula* will be found beneficial in relieving pain and clearing the eye of discharge. It quickly promotes healing when used in a strength of one in ten.

4. Keratitis – Inflammation of the Cornea. This condition is commonly associated with conjunctivitis and has the same basic etiology. There are various forms recognised – suppurative and spotted. In the vascular form small blood vessels are prominent, while the suppurative form results in the formation of ulcers or abscesses in the cornea. The spotted form is more commonly associated with a simple corneal opacity.

SYMPTOMS

Pain is a constant feature, associated with lachrymation, closure of eyelids and photophobia. Blood vessels are prominent in the vascular form extending inwards from the conjunctiva.

TREATMENT

Aurum metallicum 30c Vascular keratitis, along with extreme aversion to light. Dose: night and morning for one week.

Kali bichromicum 6c Ulceration occurs, leading to a ropy, stringy yellow discharge. Signs of pain are slight. Dose: night and morning for five days.

Conium 30c Corneal ulceration with signs of pain. Associated paralysis of ocular muscles. Dose: night and morning for one week.

Silicea 200c Neglected cases. This remedy will heal ulceration and help to absorb scar tissue. It will also help to clear any remaining opacity. Dose: once daily for one week.

5. Corneal Opacity. This is a frequent accompaniment to keratitis. It may also arise as a sequel to ophthalmia or from injury of various kinds.

SYMPTOMS

There is a general haziness of the cornea, or it may assume a mottled appearance due to irregular distribution of opaque material. When injury is the cause the resulting opacity is sharply defined and intensely white.

TREATMENT

Silicea 200c   Helps to promote absorption of opaque material. Dose: one dose per week for four weeks.

Arnica 30c   Condition resulting from injury. Dose: one dose per day for three days.

Calcarea carbonica 200c   Accompanying ulceration and a mottled cornea. Dose: once daily for one week.

Calcarea fluorica 30c   Accompanying conjunctivitis and involvement of corneal blood vessels, making the cornea reddish and muddy. Dose: night and morning for one week.

Causticum 30c   Accompanying blepharitis and tendency to cataract. Dose: night and morning for one week.

Cannabis sativa 6c   Respiratory distress, with strangury. Mucus and pus in urine. Dose: three times daily for three days.

Externally the daily application of *Cineraria* lotion will be extremely helpful.

6. **Iritis.**   Inflammation of the iris may affect the choroid and ciliary body. It is usually the result of toxins circulating in the blood as a result of bacterial disease, e.g. influenza. It is also a common sequel to periodic ophthalmia.

SYMPTOMS

Discolouration of the iris is a prominent sign, the structure assuming a dark, yellow appearance. It is accompanied by inflammation of the whole eye. Opacity of the aqueous humour occurs. Adhesions occur between the iris and the lens. Like periodic ophthalmia the condition tends to recur.

TREATMENT

Cinnabaris 6c   Redness pervades the whole eye after initial inflammation. There may be redness of mouth and throat with ulceration. Dose: night and morning for five days.

Euphrasia 6c   This good general remedy relieves pain, clears the eye of mucus or discharge. Lachrymation is acrid, thick and creamy. Dose: three times daily for five days.

Mercurius corrosivus 6c   Severe pain, worse at night. There may be slimy blood-stained diarrhoea and the eye discharge is thin, acrid and greenish. Dose: three times daily for three days.

Rhus toxicodendron 30c   Eyelids prominently swollen with surrounding cellulitis. Useful when condition results from exposure to damp for long periods. Dose: three times daily for five days.

7. Cataract. This consists of opacity of the crystalline lens or its capsule or the two together. It more frequently attacks the lens. The opacity may be complete or partial. Capsular cataract is usually dependent on injury and comes on quickly. Lenticular cataract is progressive and seen more frequently in older animals. It is also more resistant to treatment.

SYMPTOMS
An opaque body of whitish grey colour appears behind the pupil and is best seen when the pupil is dilated.

TREATMENT
Silicea 200c   Fibrous or scar tissue, which this remedy will help to absorb. Especially useful when there is accompanying corneal ulceration. Dose: once a week for four weeks.
Argentum nitricum 30c   When condition results from acute ophthalmia. Dose: once daily for two weeks.
Natrum muriaticum 200c   Slowly developing cases associated with wasting and thirst consequent on a chronic nephritis. Dose: once daily for two weeks.
Naphthaline 6c   Retinitis and corneal opacity. Dose: night and morning for one week.
Phosphorus 200c   Very white opacity and periorbital oedema. Symptoms of liver disturbance may be present. Dose: once daily for one week.
Externally an application of *Cineraria* lotion will help, but it has to be continued for some considerable time.

8. Ophthalmia. This term implies inflammation of all the structures within the eye. It usually takes the form of a suppurative process.

SYMPTOMS
There is a discharge of purulent material from one or both eyes, associated with signs of toxaemia. There may be head shaking and aversion to light. Febrile symptoms invariably present.

TREATMENT

Aconite 6c   Early febrile stage. Dose: hourly for four doses.

Belladonna 200c   Symptoms of central nervous system involvement, such as head shaking, excitement and nervousness. Pulse full and bounding, skin hot and shiny. Dose: two hourly for four doses.

Kali hydriodicum 200c   Lachrymation and discharge. This remedy, given in time, often prevents the disease process becoming established. Dose: night and morning for four days.

Silicea 200c   Corneal opacity. Suppurative states. Dose: once daily for one week.

Mercurius corrosivus 200c   Eye assumes a reddish brown appearance. There may be a purulent discharge of a greenish colour and a slimy diarrhoea. Dose: night and morning for one week.

Argentum Nitricum 30c   Profuse purulent discharge with corneal opacity and ulceration. The associated ciliary muscles are weak. Dose: night and morning for one week.

Rhus toxicodendron 1M   Orbital cellulitis and skin irritation. Muscular stiffness and erythematous sore throat may be present. Dose: once daily for one week.

Pulsatilla 30c   Purulent discharge is thick, acrid, creamy. Agglutination of eyelids. Engorgement of eye veins. Dose: night and morning for one week.

Hepar sulphuris 200c   Excess of purulent discharge. Lower potencies will hasten this, while the higher will hasten resolution. Dose: night and morning for a week.

9.   Periodic Ophthalmia.   This is a specific form of ophthalmia, so called because of its recurrent or relapsing nature. It is more frequent in male than female animals and in the young subject rather than the old.

SYMPTOMS

Early signs include slight lachrymation and a gradual involvement, or more sudden appearances with profuse discharge. Extreme sensitivity to light accompanies these symptoms. The conjunctiva is red and swollen and there are febrile symptoms. The cornea gradually becomes whitish or opaque. The main peculiarity of this condition is that favourable cases show relapse and lead to a repetition of the symptoms. The disease may spread from one eye to the other and each attack leaves the eyes more damaged.

TREATMENT
The animal should immediately be placed in a darkened stall or loose-box, to avoid exposure to light.

Aconitum napellus 6x and Belladonna 200c   These two remedies should be given at hourly intervals in alternation with each other, for four doses each.

Kali bichromicum 200c   Discharge tough and stringy and is a deep yellow colour. Dose: night and morning for one week.

Conium 30c   Excessive photophobia and lachrymation. Paralysis or weakness of eye muscles. Dose: night and morning for one week.

Graphites 6c   Intolerance of light, especially artificial light. Eyelids red and fissured, with sticky discharge. Dose: three times daily for one week.

Silicea 200c   This remedy will hasten resolution of scar tissue which may remain after damage by inflammation and ulceration. Dose: once daily for one week, followed by one dose weekly of potency 1M for four weeks.

10. Hydrophthalmia.   This term is used to denote a general dilation of the structures of the eye, causing an increase in volume. It is seen occasionally in the horse.

SYMPTOMS
The entire eye increases markedly in size and there is excessive tension on palpitation. This leads to dilation of blood vessels, especially veins leading to oedema.

TREATMENT
Apis 6c   This remedy will hasten resorption of fluid and reduces tension in the eyeball. Dose: three times daily for four days.

Osmium 6c   Increase in intraocular tension. Pain and lachrymation. Dose: three times daily for five days.

Physostigma 6c   Profuse lachrymation accompanies a paresis of ciliary muscles. Contraction of pupils and photophobia. Dose: night and morning for one week.

Gelsemium 200c   Heaviness of eyelids, with twitching of orbital muscles. There is a generalised inflammation of the serous structures of the eye. Dose: once daily for one week.

Phosphorus 200c   Accompanying retinitis and periorbital oedema. Dose: night and morning for one week.

11. Dacryocystitis — Inflammation of the Lachrymal Sac.

This condition may be acute or chronic. It may be associated with a conjunctivitis or catarrhal condition of the nasal passages. It may follow an attack of strangles.

SYMPTOMS

Profuse lachrymation is an early sign, followed by a prominent swelling in the inner canthus of the eye, caused by distention of the sac. A lachrymal fistula may arise if the sac ruptures.

TREATMENT

Iodun 6c Acute cases with dilation of pupils. Eyeballs are in constant motion. The animal may have a weathered appearance of the skin. Profuse lachrymation. Dose: night and morning for one week.

Silicea 200c Swelling of the sac is accompanied by a similar condition of the duct. There may be an associated ulceration of cornea. Dose: once daily for five days.

Fluoric acid 30c Associated lachrymal fistula. Dose: one night and morning for two weeks.

Natrum muriaticum 200c Tendency to stricture of the lachrymal duct. Dose: once daily for ten days.

III Affections of the Ear

1. **Pus in the Guttural Pouch.**   This may arise from an accompanying inflammation of the pharynx, or as a result of spread from a neighbouring abscess. It is sometimes seen as a sequel to strangles. If not treated adequately in the acute stage, the condition becomes chronic.

SYMPTOMS
A nasal discharge first appears, seen especially when the head is lowered during grazing. The character of the discharge is thin and liquid, yellowish-white in colour. There is an accompanying swelling of the submaxillary and partoid glands which become firm and tender. There is difficulty in swallowing and respiration may be interfered with in severe cases.

TREATMENT
Hepar sulphuris 6x − 200c   When used in the lower potencies, this remedy will hasten discharge of purulent material, while in higher potency it will help to resorb the condition. Dose: three times daily for two days of lower potencies. One dose night and morning for four days of the higher potency. This is the chief remedy in the acute condition.
Silicea 200c   A suitable remedy for the less acute condition. The discharge it whitish and purulent. It will help to promote healing of ulcerated surfaces within the pouch. Dose: once daily for seven days.
Hydrastis 30c   This remedy is indicated if the discharge takes the form of a simple catarrh without purulent involvement. Dose: three times daily for two days.
Mercurius corrosivus 200c   The indications for this remedy are greenish coloured thin purulent discharge, possibly blood-stained. This may accompany salivation and slimy diarrhoea. Dose: three times daily for three days.

Kali bichromicum 30c   Pus bright yellow and stringy. Dose: once daily for one week.

2.   Tympanitis of the Guttural Pouch.   Foals between the ages of two months and one year have been known to suffer from this condition. It is caused by the accumulation of air in the pouch, which cannot then escape because of a blockage in the Eustachian tube. It is usually bilateral.

SYMPTOMS
The parotid region becomes the seat of a painless elastic swelling, giving resonance on percussion. The swelling may extend downwards to include the throat region and when this happens interference with respiration and swallowing occurs.

TREATMENT
Calcarea carbonica 200c   This remedy is associated with an accompanying ear discharge, which causes eruption around the ear. Dose: once daily for one week.
Kali muriaticum 6c   Indicated when there is accompanying swelling of associated glands. There may also be catarrhal discharge from ear and nose. Dose: three times daily for three days.
Mercurius dulcis 30c   This is a useful remedy for treating blockage of the Eustachian tube, especially if associated with middle ear discharge. Dose: three times daily for four days.
Pulsatilla 30c   Indicated when the ear becomes swollen, discharging a bland mucous catarrh. Dose: night and morning for four days.

IV Affections of the Nervous System

1. **Encephalitis.**   This term implies inflammation of the brain, or any inflammatory lesion occurring in brain tissue. It leads to loss of nervous function.

SYMPTOMS
Encephalitis is usually accompanied by fever and toxaemia; anorexia, depression and tachycardia occur also. Normal stimuli produce exaggerated responses, the animal being easily startled. There may be convulsions, accompanied by squinting of eyes and clamping of jaws. Paresis and ataxia may precede paralysis.

TREATMENT
Aconitum napellus 6c   If seen early enough, should be given in the febrile stage. Dose: hourly for four doses.
Belladonna 1M   This is a very useful remedy. There is an accompanying full bounding pulse, dilated pupils and a smooth hot skin. Dose: hourly for four doses.
Stramonium 30c   Indicated when signs of vertigo appear, such as a tendency to stagger and fall sideways. The eyes are usually wide open and staring. Dose: four times daily for two days.
Hyoscyamus 200c   Indications for this remedy include frequent head shaking and a tendency to muscular twitchings. There may be signs of abdominal discomfort. Dose: three times daily for three days.
Phosphorus 200c   This is a useful remedy in less acute cases, showing a tendency to recur. The animal becomes unsteady after rising. Dose: night and morning for one week.
Aethusa 30c   Indicated when there is accompanying photophobia and acute abdominal symptoms, e.g. the passing of flatus which gives relief to the head symptoms. Dose: three times daily for three days.
Camphora 6c   Indicated when the body surface becomes cold

and there is a tendency to collapse. A watery stool may accompany the condition. Dose: two hourly for four doses.

Cuprum aceticum 6c   The indications for this remedy are violent tenesmus and the passage of a slimy brown stool. Respirations are difficult and the animal moves the tongue in and out of the mouth frequently. Dose: three hourly for four doses.

Solanum nigrum 30c   Associated with coryza and eye symptoms such as alternate dilations and contractions of pupils. Dose: three times daily for three days.

Zincum metallicum 6c   Indicated when there is a tendency for the head to roll from side to side. Hyperaesthesia and hyperexcitability are present. Dose: three times daily for three days.

2. Meningitis.   Inflammation of the meninges is usually secondary to bacterial or viral disease.

SYMPTOMS

This condition is characterised by fever and muscle rigidity. Sensitivity of the skin is a common symptom. Trismus and opisthotonus may occur. There is retraction of the head and stiffness of neck muscles. Paresis of hindquarters is common.

TREATMENT

Aconitum napellus 6c   Should be given in the early febrile stage. The animal usually looks anxious and there is a rapid, short pulse. Dose: hourly for four hours.

Apis 6c   This remedy is indicated if the condition in the nerve stage is accompanied by oedema of the meninges. Dose: every two hours for four doses.

Belladonna 1M   The indications for this remedy are an accompanying encephalitis, with dilated pupils and a throbbing pulse. The skin is smooth and hot; sweating is common. Dose: two hourly for three doses.

Helleborus niger 6c   Indicated when there are signs of considerable pain. The animal bores the head against any convenient object. Dose: two hourly for four doses.

Zincum metallicum 6c   Useful when the animal is easily startled. Rolling of the head is a common symptom. Paddling of the feet may occur. Dose: three times daily for three days.

Cicuta virosa 200c   Indicated where there is contraction of neck muscles and the head is twisted to one side. There is a tendency to stare fixedly and to squint. Dose: three times daily for three days.

Laburnum 6c   Useful when the spinal, as well as the cerebral, meninges are affected. There is difficulty in moving the fore feet and twitching of the facial muscles occurs. Unequal dilation of pupils is a common symptom. Dose: three times daily for three days.

Bryonia 6c   Indicated in cases showing vertigo. The animal resents movement and there is excessive dryness of mucous membranes e.g. seen in the mouth, where the lips show a parched appearance and there is great thirst. Dose: three times daily for three days.

Agaricus muscarius 200c   Useful in spinal meningitis showing a tendency to paralysis of the lower limbs. This is accompanied by twitching and vertigo which is accentuated in bright light. Dose: three times daily for four days.

Lathyrus sativa 6c   Indicated also in spinal meningitis with an accompanying myelitis. Movements are weak and tottering with muscle rigidity. Reflexes are increased and there is a tendency to emaciation of gluteal muscles. Dose: three times daily for three days.

Strychninum 200c   Indicated when there is violent jerking and twitching of muscles and opisthotonus. The limbs become stiff. Dose: three times daily for three days.

3.   **Paralysis of the Facial Nerve.**   This is of fairly common occurrence in the horse and may be unilateral, or bilateral. There are various causes, including traumatism and exposure to cold. A toxic form may arise as a sequel to some infectious disease, such as strangles or influenza.

SYMPTOMS

When the condition is unilateral, the lips are drawn towards the sound side. Bilateral involvement precludes grasping of food, while the lower lip hangs down. There is also difficulty in drinking. Occasionally the animal has difficulty in closing the eyelids.

TREATMENT

Gelsemium 200c   This is one of the main remedies in treating motor paralysis of various groups of muscles and nerves. It is especially useful if the paralysis is a sequel to infectious disease, particularly influenza. Dose: once daily for one week. It may be necessary to continue treatment with higher potencies.

Causticum 30c   This remedy is particularly useful if the condition has arisen as a result of exposure to cold. Dose: night and morning for five days.

Ammonium phosphoricum 6c   A lesser known remedy which should be remembered when there is an accompanying early morning coryza. Dose: night and morning for five days.

Zincum picricum 6c   Indicated in chorea-like twitchings of facial muscles together with general weakness and debility. Dose: night and morning for one week.

V Diseases of Respiratory Tract

1.   Epistaxis – Nose Bleed.   This condition may arise from injuries or over-exertion in which case the blood is usually bright red, but it can also be a symptom of various diseases, e.g. influenza or pneumonia and may also be associated with ulceration of the nasal mucosa. In diseased conditions, the blood is usually discoloured. Slight bleeding may stop of its own accord, but when it is excessive, it demands immediate attention. When the bleeding is the result of constitutional illness, the underlying condition must be remembered when considering symptoms.

TREATMENT

Aconitum napellus 6c   Bleeding results from over-exertion, and immediate treatment is advisable. Dose: every hour for four doses.

Arnica 30c   Local injuries causing the nose-bleed. Dose: every four hours for three doses. Externally, the remedy should be given in tincture or liniment form by plugging the nostril with cotton wool soaked in tincture.

Ammonium carb. 6c   Fat subjects, if the condition is dependent on constitutional upset. Dose: every three hours for four doses.

Belladonna 1M   Feverish state, showing involvement of the central nervous system. Full pulse, dilated pupils and sweating. Symptoms relieved by keeping patient in a loose-box from which the light has been excluded. Dose: hourly for four doses.

Bryonia 6c   Constitutional cases showing early morning bleeding. Animal better at rest. Dose: three times daily for three days.

China off. 30c   After severe bleeding, great weakness. Dose: every four hours for four doses.

Hamamelis 6c   Passive bleeding of dark non-coagulated blood. Throat veins engorged. Dose: three times daily for three days.

Ferrum phos. 6c   Animal nervous and sensitive, blood bright red. Dose: every three hours for three doses.

Ficus religiosa 1x   Accompanying bleeding from lungs, general respiratory distress. Dose: four times daily for two days.

Ipecacuanha 30c   Over-eating and digestive upsets. Blood bright red. Dose: every four hours for four doses.

Melilotus 6c   Muscular weakness. Nose may have polypi leading to haemorrhage which is usually profuse. Dose: three times daily for three days.

Millefolium 6c   Blood bright red, but there may also be blood from bowels or kidneys. Persistent high temperature. Dose: every two hours for four doses.

2.   Coryza.   Inflammation of the nasal mucous membranes may arise from exposure to cold or damp and frequently attacks horses that are in poor condition or badly housed. Coryza has a tendency to extend to the laryngeal and lower respiratory areas leading to a possible bronchitis or pneumonia.

SYMPTOMS

Early signs include sneezing and swelling of eyelids, followed by a thin mucous discharge from the nose. Discharge soon becomes thick and catarrhal. Most cases resolve quickly, but a chronic form may supervene in poorly nourished animals. Laryngitis and cough may accompany the condition, the former being associated with throat swelling.

TREATMENT

The patient should be put in a clean, well-ventilated loose-box and consideration given to the following remedies:-

Aconitum 6c   Early stages, when mucous membrane of the nose is dry and hot. Animal thirsty and feverish. Dose: hourly for four doses.

Arsenicum alb 1M   Discharge is acrid. Swollen eyelids, thirst for small quantities. Restless, worse after midnight. Dose: every two hours for four doses.

Allium cepa 6c   Discharge bland, watery. Eyes red, showing lachrymation and photophobia. Dose: hourly for four doses.

Hepar sulphuris 200c   Sneezing, with ulceration of nostrils. Discharge thick and purulent, foul-smelling. Sensitive to pain, resenting cold wind. Dose: three times daily for two days.

Natrum muriaticum 1M   Discharge whitish, albuminous-looking. There may be violent sneezing. Dose: every two hours for four doses.

Hydrastis 30c   Discharge catarrhal and bland. Dose: three times daily for two days.

Kali bichromicum 200c   Discharge chronic, tends to become thick and tough. Dose: night and morning for five days.

Mercurius dulcis 6c   Throat involved, nasal discharge greenish and thin. Dose: four times daily for one day.

Silicea 200c   Discharge thin, greyish, associated with caries of nasal septum and neighbouring structures. Crusts form inside nose. Dose: once daily for six days.

3.   Nasal Gleet.   This term implies a chronic discharge caused by a catarrhal or purulent inflammation of long standing, which may extend to the facial sinuses.

SYMPTOMS

A copious purulent secretion appears in one or both nostrils. The character of the discharge varies from thin and mucoid to thick and purulent and may be accompanied by swelling and tenderness of the sub-maxilliary glands.

TREATMENT

Kali bichromicum 200c   Secretion thick and lumpy, difficult to expel from the nostrils. Dose: night and morning for five days.

Hydrastis 30c   Discharge catarrhal and non-purulent. Dose: three times daily for three days.

Mercurius corrosivus 200c   Associated with disease of nasal bones. Discharge is purulent, greenish, sometimes streaked with blood. Dose: night and morning for four days.

Balsam of Peru 6c   Discharge thick and foetid, frequently accompanied by catarrhal discharge elsewhere. Dose: three times daily for two days.

Pulsatilla 30c   Greenish scales in nostrils, associated with catarrhal discharge, often worse in morning. Dose: three times daily for three days.

4.   Ozaena.   This is a form of nasal gleet producing symptoms like ordinary gleet, but with an extremely foul-smelling discharge.

TREATMENT

Cadmium sulph 30c   Nasal polypi, with ulceration and obstruction. Dose: three times daily for three days.

Aurum metallicum 30c   Extremely offensive odour with purulent bloody discharge. Nose swollen, discharge worse at night. Dose: three times daily for four days.

Lemna minor 30c   Nasal polypi and swollen turbinate bones. Worse in wet weather. Putrid smell from discharge. Dose: three times daily for three days.

Asafoetida 6c   Very offensive purulent discharge. There may be caries of nasal bones. Dose: three times daily for four days.

Mercurius corrosivus 200c   Perforation of nasal septum accompanied by a greenish thin discahrge which may be blood-stained. Dose: night and morning for three days.

5.   Pus in the Facial Sinuses.   Catarrhal conditions of the upper respiratory tract may involve the sinuses, leading to a chronic sinusitis.

SYMPTOMS

There is a discharge of pus from the nostrils, with swelling over the nasal bones and maxillary region. Dullness on percussion is seen over the affected area.

TREATMENT

As an alternative to surgical intervention, the following remedies should be considered:-

Hepar sulphuris 200c   Sensitivity to draughts and cold. Extreme sensitivity to touch or pressure on the affected area. Dose: night and morning for one week.

Hydrastis 30c   Pus bland, flowing freely from nostrils. Dose: three times daily for six days.

Mercurius corrosivus 200c   Purulent material blood-stained, greenish. Dose: night and morning for five days.

Kali bichromicum 200c   Long standing cases showing tough stringy discharge. Dose: night and morning for five days.

Silicea 200c   Chronic cases showing thin, whitish pus associated with affections of maxillary and nasal bones. Dose: night and morning for five days.

Arsenicum alb 1M   Discharge acrid, tending to excoriate the nostrils. Restless, worse after midnight. Dose: once daily for five days.

6.   Laryngitis.   The larynx may become inflamed, accompanied by secretion of mucus which may be profuse enough to interfere with the animal's breathing. It is frequently an accompaniment of catarrhal conditions or infections such as strangles or influenza.

SYMPTOMS

Breathing is quickened and attended by rough snoring sound and harsh cough which can be increased by pressure on the larynx. Breathing becomes more laboured when oedema of the glottis becomes profuse. The swelling and oedema appear on the anterior of the throat.

TREATMENT

Aconitum napellus 6c   Early stages, febrile signs such as quickened pulse and respiration. Dose: hourly for four doses.

Apis 6c   Oedema prominent symptom, throat becoming soft and swollen. Dose: three times daily for two days.

Spongia tosta 6c   Severe attacks, with characteristic cough. Dose: three times daily for three days.

Belladonna 1M   Inflammation extends to pharyngeal area. Difficulty in swallowing. Full bounding pulse, dilated pupils and smooth shiny skin. Dose: every two hours for four doses.

Mercurius cyanatus 30c   Rough whitish membrane covers bottom of tongue and upper laryngeal area. Salivation is increased. Dose: three times daily for three days.

Sanguinaria 6c   Threatened oedema of larynx. Cough with tenderness over wind pipe. Dose: three times daily for three days.

7.   Bronchitis.   Inflammation of the bronchial mucous membrane may arise independently of other illnesses, or may be a sequel to influenza or catarrhal states. The condition invariably involves lung tissue, being more a broncho-pneumonia than a pure bronchitis. It may arise simply by exposure to cold dry winds or to damp and cold.

SYMPTOMS

Breathing is accelerated, pulse becomes full and quick, accompanied by a frequent painful cough. Mucous secretion soon becomes purulent and may run from the nose as well as appear in the cough. Rattling respiratory sounds can be heard over the rib area.

TREATMENT

Aconitum napellus 6c   Early stages, with hot, dry skin, feverish symptoms, and anxious expression. Dose: hourly for four doses.

Belladonna 1M   Pulse full and bounding, with dilated pupils, sweating and excitement. Dose: every two hours for four doses.

Antimonium tartiaricum 30c   Moist cough with threatened pulmonary oedema. Rattling sounds may be heard in the chest, respirations increased. Dose: three times daily for three days.

Bryonia 6c   Cough hard and dry, pleura become affected. Relief from pressure over ribs. Dose: three times daily for three days.

Dulcamara 6c   Condition has origin in damp surroundings and coughing worse after exertion. Dose: three times daily for three days.

Kali bichromicum 200c   Phlegm in bronchial tubes difficult to expel. Nasal discharge. Dose: three times daily for three days.

Drosers 6c   Coughing becomes spasmodic in character. Paroxysms follow one another rapidly. Dose: three times daily for three days.

Squilla 6c   Coughing is accompanied by fluent coryza and much sneezing. Coughing produces slimy expectoration, brought on by drinking or exertion of any kind. Dose: three times daily for four days.

Arsenicum iodatum 6c   Chronic cases with periods of quiescence alternating with bouts of coughing. Very useful remedy for bronchial conditions which fail to clear properly. Dose: night and morning for four days.

Spongia 6c   Bouts of coughing eased by eating or drinking, worse by exposure to cold air. Dose: three times daily for four doses.

Sulphur 30c   Give as a constitutional remedy when recovery takes place. Dose: once daily for five days.

8. Pulmonary Congestion.   The term implies a sudden engorgement of the lungs and may occur after severe or long-continued exertion.

SYMPTOMS

Breathing is oppressed and laboured, nostrils become flayed in the effort to inhale. The pulse is strong and full and may reach ninety beats per minute. Occasionally blood may come from the nose. Legs and ears become cold and the eyes betray anxiety.

TREATMENT

Aconitum napellus 6c   A preliminary remedy, as soon as condition is suspected. Dose: hourly for four doses.

Ammonium caust. 6c   Increase in mucus and moist coughing, with exhaustion and muscular weakness. Dose: three times daily for three days.

Belladonna 200c   Hot dry skin, dilated pupils and excitability. Pulse full and bounding. Dose: every two hours for four doses.

Ferrum phos. 6c   Blood is coughed up and condition decreases in severity as night approaches. Dose: three times daily for three days.

Veratrum viride 6c   Congestion accompanied by scanty urine, rapid pulse of low tension. Dose: three times daily for two days.

Apis 30c   Pulmonary oedema severe, accompanied by extension of oedema to the laryngeal area. Dose: night and morning for four days.

9.   Pleurisy.   Injuries to the chest may lead to pleurisy and it may also arise from exposure to cold and damp.

SYMPTOMS

A quick, thready pulse precedes a bout of shivering. Signs of pain over the chest are indicated by abdominal breathing. There are general febrile symptoms such as discolouration of the conjunctiva and quickened pulse. The expression is anxious. Inspiration is difficult, but expiration is accomplished without much trouble. Cough is short, dry and hacking, with pain. Pressure over the ribs causes resentment. Sometimes the skin over the pleural area becomes thickened into folds. Occasionally oedema of the pleural cavities occurs leading to increased respiratory distress.

TREATMENT

Aconitum napellus 6c   The early febrile stage. Dose: hourly for four doses.

Bryonia 30c   Better at rest. Pressure over pleural area relieves. Cough usually hard and dry. Dose: every two hours for four doses.

Apis 30c   Oedema occurs in pleural cavities, urine scanty and high-coloured. Dose: three times daily for three days.

Cantharis 200c   Pleural effusion. Mucus expectorated with cough is usually blood-stained. Severe straining when trying to pass urine. Dose: three times daily for two days.

Guaiacum 6c   Articular surfaces of ribs more sensitive to pain than elsewhere. This may not be easy to diagnose, but coughing relieves the symptoms and expectoration eases the shortness of respiration. Dose: three times daily for two days.

Kali carbonicum 200c   Symptoms of pain worse on right side. Cough worse in early morning and there is usually a dry throat. Dose: three times daily for three days.

Senega 30c   In older animals, sneezing occurs after coughing. Useful also in exudative pleurisy. Dose: three times daily for three days.

Squilla 6c   Coughing provoked by drinking. Pain extends to abdominal muscles. Increased urination towards evening. Dose: three times daily for two days.

Arsenicum iodatum 30c   Chronic state, with persistent dry cough remaining after treatment. Useful generally for cases slow to respond or heal. Dose: once daily for one week.

Sulphur 30c   Use in the convalescent stage of pleurisy. Dose: once daily for six days.

Sanguinaria 6c   Cough raises rust-coloured sputum, with tenderness over right side. Cough always returns after each febrile attack. Dose: three times daily for three days.

10.   Influenza.   This is due to various febrile agents. In its pure state, it consists of first a fever, and secondly a specific affection of the mucous membranes of the upper respiratory tract and eyes. It most commonly affects young horses and appears usually in spring and autumn.

SYMPTOMS

Febrile signs first appear and the animal is dull and listless. There is a fast, thready pulse. Urine may be scanty and high coloured. The congestive swelling of the nose extends down the respiratory tract, giving at first a mucoid, and later a purulent, discharge. The cough is harsh and dry and breathing is accelerated. The nervous system is also affected — state of general languor and muscular weakness. The conjunctivae are discoloured yellowish-brown.

TREATMENT

Aconitum napellus 6c   Early stage when febrile signs accompany anxious expression. Dose: every hour for four hours.

Belladonna 200c or 1M   Acute cases, with full pulse, dilated pupils. Skin hot and shiny. Excitement and head-shaking. Dose: every hour for four doses.

Gelsemium 1M   Langour, muscular weakness, incoordination of movement. Dose: every two hours for four doses.

Bryonia 6c   Harsh, dry cough. Pleuritic symptoms such as pain over chest and friction sounds are heard on ausculation. Relief on pressure. Short, grunting breathing. Dose: three times daily for three days.

Antimonium tartaricum 30c   Saliva appears accompanied by moist cough and the presence of mucous rales on auscultation. Dose: night and morning for four days.

Phosphorus 200c   Breathing short and rapid, pneumonia threatened. Dose: three times daily for two days.

Lycopodium 200c   Once pneumonia has set in and animal shows laboured movement of the alae nasi, independent of respiration. Dose: three times daily for two days.

Arsenicum alb. 1M   Symptoms generally worse towards or after midnight. Animal restless, drinks frequent small quantities. Skin dry and staring. Dose: every two hours for four doses.

Nux vomica 6c   Constipation and capricious appetite. Dose: every three hours for four doses.

Ammonium caust. 6c   Pulmonary congestion supervenes, oedema threatens, with coldness of skin. Dose: three times daily for three days.

11.   Pneumonia.   Inflammation of the lung tissue may appear as a result of overwork or chill. It is also a sequel to disease such as influenza or bronchitis.

SYMPTOMS

Frequent pulse rate, with discoloured conjunctivae, followed by laboured breathing and anxious or distressed look. As the condition progresses heaving on the flanks takes place and neck becomes extended as the animal seeks to take in more air. Legs and ears become cold and the mucous membranes of nose and mouth assume a dusky dark bluish tinge. Cough may be blood-stained or rust-coloured containing shreds of fibrin in the mucus.

TREATMENT

Aconitum napellus 6c   Should always be given first. Dose: every half-hour for six doses.

Bryonia 6c   Cough hard and dry and pleurisy is severe. Worse on movement and pressure over chest relieves. Dose: three times daily for two days.

Antimonium tartaricum 30c   Rattling of mucus, accumulation of frothy saliva. Dose: three times daily for three days.

Lycopodium 200c   Cases showing rapid wasting and involvement of the alae nasi. Dose: every two hours for four doses.

Phosphorus 200c   A main remedy, once hepatisation has set in. Pressure resented, particularly over left side. Sputum rust-coloured. Trembling of body. Dose: every two hours for four doses.

Iodum 30c   Hepatisation spreads rapidly, full pulse, absence of pain over chest. Temperature remains high, sputum blood-streaked. Dose: every hour for four doses.

Sanguinaria 30c   Heart symptoms such as valvular weakness appear and signs of accompanying pulmonary congestion set in. Urine may contain phosphates. Dose: night and morning for five days.

Tuberculinium aviare 200c.   Chiefly for young foals with loss of strength and appetite. The apices of the lungs are more involved than other portions of lung tissue. Dose: night and morning for five days.

Sulphur 30c   Expectoration becomes greenish and purulent. Pulse rate decreases towards evening and rises again later in the evening. Dose: three times daily for three days.

Beryllium 30c   Dyspnoea out of proportion to clinical findings. Also associated with skin symptoms. Dose: three times daily for three days.

12. **Cough**. While coughing is frequently associated with various pulmonary infections, it may arise as a seemingly independent syndrome, and takes various forms:-

1 Pleuritic cough. Short and dry and the animal shows pain when coughing.
2 Bronchitic cough. Starts dry and frequent, becomes moist and soft.
3 Pneumonic cough. Frequent, may contain rust-coloured fibrinous deposits in sputum.
4 Simple Catarrhal cough. Usually moist and infrequent.
5 Stomach or intestinal cough. Various forms. Dependent on alimentary disorders.

TREATMENT

Bryonia 6c Pleuritic cough, dry, symptoms worse on movement. Better from pressure, or pressure over affected area. Dose: three times daily for three days.

Arsenicum iodatum 6c Cough lingers after chest infections such as influenza or bronchitis. Dose: three times daily for three days.

Belladonna 30c Cough accompanied by full pulse, hot smooth skin, dilated pupils, nervous symptoms. Dose: every two hours for four doses.

Drosera 6c Spasmodic cough of chronic nature. Sometimes associated with asthmatic symptoms, worse early morning. Dose: three times daily for three days.

Nux vomica 6c Origin in digestive upsets. Dose: three times daily for three days.

Causticum 30c Cough relieved by drinking. Expectorations scanty. Dose: night and morning for four days.

Arsenicum alb. 1M Cough worse after midnight, animal restless, thirsty with dry skin. Cough worse after drinking, even small quantities. Dose: night and morning for five days.

Spongia 30c Cough worse on inspiration and worse towards midnight. Relieved by drinking. Sometimes associated with heart disease. Dose: night and morning for three days.

Sticta 6c Cough originates more in the trachea, is worse in evening and during the night and on inspiration. Dose: three times daily for three days.

Stannum 30c Cough accompanies established influenza. Worse in latter part of the day. Expectoration forcibly expelled. Dose: three times daily for three days.

VI Diseases of the Circulatory System

1. **Tachycardia.** This is the name given to an increased heart rhythm and may be brought about by a fall in arterial blood-pressure, or by influences leading to pain and excitement. An independent form called paroxysmal tachycardia sometimes occurs in the horse. Disease of heart muscle may cause this form.

SYMPTOMS
The pulse is small and the heart sounds are increased. Exercise is poorly tolerated.

TREATMENT
Crataegus 6c   This is very useful in the paroxysmal form to help restore strength to the heart muscle. Dose: four times daily for one week.

Lycopus 6c   Indicated where there is palpitation from nervous excitement. Pulse is tremulous and weak. There may be passive haemorrhages. Dose: three times daily for four or five days.

Convallaria 6c   Indicated in venous stasis and dyspnoea. Even slight exertion brings on palpitation. Pulse is very irregular and rapid. Dose: three times daily for five days.

Strophanthus 6c   An irregular pulse, associated with myocard-itis, will benefit from this remedy. The animal may show signs of pain on movement. Dose: three times daily for three days.

Aconitum napellus 6c   Pain over left shoulder region, pulse full and tense, strained anxious expression. Dose: three times daily for four days.

Iberis 6c   Palpitation accompanied by choking symptoms and an irregular, intermittent pulse. Palpitation easily induced. Dose: two hourly for four doses.

Lilium tigrinum 30c Palpitation and very rapid pulse, associated with frequent urination, the urine being whitish and hot. There is also urging to defaecate and stool may be blood-stained and contain mucus. Dose: every two hours for four doses.

Naja 6c Irregular pulse of low tension, associated with lethargy and threatened paralysis. Palpitation is common. Dose: every three hours for four doses.

Phosphorus 30c When this remedy is needed, there is violent palpitation. The pulse is weak and soft. Liver symptoms may be prominent giving tenderness over the hepatic region. Stools are clay-coloured and there may be purpura-like haemorrhages on mucous membranes and skin. Dose: three times daily for four days.

Thyroidinum 6c Indicated when there is a weak, thready pulse and palpitation. The animal seldom lies down, due to numbness of lower front limbs. Pain is shown on movement and there may be a tendency to exophthalmos. Dose: three times daily for five days.

2. **Bradycardia.** This term implies slowness of heart rhythm and is often due to some extraneous cause such as increase in blood-pressure. The heart muscle is invariably sound.

SYMPTOMS

The heart's action is heavy and slow.

TREATMENT

Abies nigra 30c When there is dyspnoea with choking sounds in the throat. Coughing is frequent. Dose: three times daily for four days.

Veratrum viride 6c Pulse of low tension may be felt prominently in any superficial vessel. Respiratory symptoms include dyspnoea and congestion of the lungs. Dose: three times daily for three days.

Opium 1M Somnolent state, accompanied by severe constipation and stertorous breathing. Body surface usually very hot. Dose: three times daily for three days.

Gelsemium 200c Slow pulse with spasmodic movements of the throat muscles leading to difficulty in swallowing. Respiratory symptoms prominent. Dose: night and morning for four days.

Aesculus 6c   Abdominal discomfort such as liver dysfunction. Heart's action full and heavy. Urinary symptoms also prominent, e.g. dark and scanty. Dose: three times daily for three days.

Kalmia 6c   Pulse weak and slow with muscular stiffness, especially over lumbar region. Shoulders may also show stiffness. Dose: three times daily for three days.

Apocynum 6c   Valvular incompetence and dusky appearance of visible mucous membranes. Dose: three times daily for five to six days.

3.   Pericarditis.   Inflammation of the heart sac is rarely met with as a primary condition and is invariably a sequel to some bacterial or viral infection, such as influenza, and frequently follows pleurisy.

SYMPTOMS
The pulse becomes hard and wiry and is accompanied by febrile involvement. Pressure over the cardiac area causes resentment. Auscultation reveals a friction sound which ceases once effusion takes place into the pericardial sac. Fibrinous deposits may occur on the heart muscle leading to embarrassment of the heart's action. The friction sounds differ from those of pleurisy in that the latter are synchronous with respiratory movements while the former are independent of these and confined to the left chest-wall. The gait shows abduction with abdominal respiration.

TREATMENT
The animal should be isolated in a cool, well ventilated loose-box.

Aconitum napellus 6c   Should be given as early as possible in the initial febrile stage. Dose: every hour for four doses.

Bryonia 30c   Relief from pressure over the affected area. There may be a dry cough as a sequel to pleurisy. Dose: night and morning for three days.

Apis 30c   This is one of the main remedies if effusion has occurred into the pericardial sac, indicated by absence of friction sounds. Dose: night and morning for one week.

Arsenicum alb. 1M   Restlessness and prostration, with thirst for small quantities. Symptoms worse after midnight. Dose: night and morning for one week.

Spigelia 30c   Trembling pulse, animal tends to lie on right side. Great distress from movement. Dose: night and morning for five days.

Colchicum 6c   Low-tension pulse, thirst and flatulence, with increased salivation. Dose: three hourly for four doses.

Natrum muriaticum 200c   Chronic state, showing wasting and increased thirst. Dose: night and morning for ten days.

Cantharis 200c   Effusion. Urinary symptoms such as strangury; bloody urine may also be present. Dose: night and morning for five days.

Spongia 6c   Hypertrophy of heart as a result of deposition of fibrinous deposits on the myocardium, leading to chronic pericarditis. Dose: three times daily for five days.

4. Myocarditis.   Inflammation of the heart muscle is often secondary to bacterial or viral infections such as strangles or infectious anaemia, or navel-ill in foals. Degenerative lesions can arise from non-infectious causes and lead to functional or physical impairment.

SYMPTOMS
The animal usually shows a disinclination for exercise on account of this leading to embarrassment of heart's action. The heart's rate is increased and there may be an increase in the actual size of the heart, leading to respiratory distress. Bradycardia is the rule. Congestive heart states may supervene leading to a generalised oedema and severe dyspnoea.

TREATMENT
Crataegus 6c   This remedy is indicated in most cases of heart muscle weakness. Exertion brings on severe breathlessness. Useful heart medicine during the course of infectious disease. Dose: three times daily for seven days.

Arsenicum iodatum 30c   Condition a sequel to influenza or other respiratory infection. Dose: night and morning for five days.

Adonis vernalis 6c   Marked venous engorgement. Cardiac dropsy. The condition may be associated with fatty degeneration of muscle. Pulse rapid and irregular. Dose: three times daily for six days.

Strophanthis 6x   Weakness of heart muscle is accompanied by quick pulse and scanty albuminous urine. Dose: three times daily for five days.

Digitalis 6c   Palpitation is brought on by the least movement. Slow, weak, intermittent pulse which quickens on movement of the animal. Dose: three times daily for seven days.

5.   Endocarditis.   This is inflammation of the membrane lining the heart cavities. It is of more frequent occurrence than pericarditis or myocarditis. It may arise as a sequel to rheumatic involvement. Most cases are bacterial in origin. It may also arise from parasitism due to strongyle infestation.

SYMPTOMS
Excitement of a febrile nature is accompanied by a small inter-mittent pulse. Body temperature may fall owing to a deficient peripheral circulation. Ulcerative lesions frequently appear on the heart valves leading to symptoms of congestive heart failure. In the horse aortic valves are usually affected, but the mitral valve may also suffer. The chief heart sound is a deep murmur varying according to which valve is affected. It frequently takes the form of a 'bellows' sound. Distension of the jugular vein may be seen.

TREATMENT
Calcarea fluorica 30c   Fibrinous deposits occur on the heart valves and this remedy hastens their absorption. Dose: night and morning for five days.

Lycopus 30c   Palpitation accompanies a weak intermittent pulse. Heart sounds are very intense. A wheezing cough may be present. Dose: night and morning for five days.

Naja 6c   Lesions occur after bacterial or viral diseases. Suitable for both acute and chronic cases. Pulse irregular and body cold. Dose: three times daily for four days.

Convallaria 6c   The pulse is extremely rapid and irregular. Venous stasis is prominent. Dose: three times daily for five days.

Adonis vernalis 6c   If rheumatic involvement is suspected, with symptoms of vertigo. Venous engorgement also suspected. Dose: three times daily for five days.

Kalmia 6c   Tumultuous heart action. Kidney involvement fre-quent. Signs of pain over left shoulder region. Dose: three times daily for one week.

Aconitum napellus 6c   Tense full pulse, pulsation of cartoid arteries; Animal appears anxious, with uneasiness and signs of pain. Dose: every two hours for five doses.

Cactus grandiflorus 6c   Mitral valve incompetence. There may be cold sweating and signs of pain on movement. Blood pressure is low and heart sounds are increased. Dose: three times daily for one week.

Spigelia 6c   Prominent dyspnoea. Animal tends to lie on right side, possibly due to pain over left shoulder area. The least movement aggravates. Dose: three times daily for four days.

6.   Valvular Disease.   Affections of the heart valves usually have their origin in endocarditis. Degenerative lesions of the aortic valves have been reported in horses. Valvular disease is diagnosed by murmurs heard on auscultation and may take the form of stenosis or incompetence.

Stenosis of Aortic Valves. This has little significance functionally unless accompanied by an abnormal pulse. The most audible sound is a harsh murmur associated with systole. It usually replaces the first heart sound and is heard posteriorly on the left side.

Incompetence of Aortic Valves. When this is sufficiently advanced, it is accompanied by a very full pulse, along with a high systolic and a low diastolic blood pressure. Sometimes the pulse may be seen in the small peripheral vessels.

Stenosis of the Mitral Valve. Passage of blood through a narrowed valve opening leads to a diastolic murmur, the duration of which being dependent on the severity of the stenosis. The murmur is most audible at the heart's apex on the left side and carries through the second heart to the beginning of the first. Incomplete filling of the left ventricle may lead to pulse changes.

Incompetence of the Mitral Valve. Leakage of blood during the heart's systole leads to a murmur heard at the apex of the heart on the left side. Normally there are no pulse changes.

Stenosis and Incompetence of Tricuspid Valve. This produces a symptom picture analogous to mitral valve affections, except that the heart murmur is found apically on the right side. A jugular pulse commonly accompanies tricuspid incompetence.

The diagnosis of these conditions depends on auscultation of the murmurs which replace normal heart sounds. These differ from pericardial friction sounds in being less audible and not differing in intensity with the heart's action.

TREATMENT

Lycopus 6c   Tumultuous heart action, accompanied by a cough which contains blood. Dose: three times daily for four days.

Naja 6c   Useful after infectious diseases, when body cold and pulse irregular. Dose: three times daily for five days.

Adonis vernalis 6c   Marked venous engorgement with asthmatic symptoms and palpitation. Dose: three times daily for five or six days.

Crataegus 6c   Weakness of heart muscle with slow, weak pulse. Dose: three times daily for six or seven days.

Spongia 6c   Valvular incompetence with breathlessness and anxious expression. Peripheral veins are prominent and there is usually a dry, hard cough. Dose: three times daily for six days.

Spigelia 6c   When rheumatic diathesis is suspected. Movement aggravates and animal lies on right side only. Pain and tenderness evident over left shoulder area. Dose: three times daily for five days.

Strophanthus 6c   Heart muscle weak. Incompetence. Urinary symptoms. Dose: three times daily for five days.

Convallaria 6c   Very rapid and irregular pulse. Dose: three times daily for seven days.

Laurocerasus 6c   Mitral incompetence. Mucous membranes of mouth and nose become cyanosed and dusky. Dose: three times daily for five days.

VII Diseases of Blood
and Blood-Forming Organs

1. Dehydration. This arises when excessive fluid loss takes place and can be caused by super-purgation, polyuria and prolonged severe sweating. Depression of tissue fluid levels takes place and leads to a reduction in the fluid content of the blood.

SYMPTOMS
The main signs are dry shrunken appearance of the external skin and a harsh appearance of the coat. The eye becomes sunken. Muscular weakness and increased thirst are apparent. Urine becomes scanty and of a high specific gravity. The heart rate is increased and blood pressure falls.

TREATMENT
China off. 30c This is the best remedy for this condition, helping to restore strength and promote a return to normal physiological condition. Dose: three times daily for three days.

2. Haemorrhage. This may take several forms, such as epistaxis, haemoptysis, metrorrhagia, haematemesis etc. and each case must be considered on its own symptomatology.

TREATMENT
Ipecacuanha 30c Useful when the blood is bright red and profuse. Dose: every hour for four doses.
Phosphorus 200c Indicated when there are extravasations of blood in the skin and mucous membranes. Purpura-like ecchymoses occur. Capillary bleeding is common. Dose: three times daily for three days.
Melilotus 6c This remedy is associated with general congestive

states. Throbbing of neck arteries is common. Dose: three days.

Ficus religiosa 6c   Indicated when there is respiratory distress. Blood is usually bright red. Dose: every three hours for four doses.

Ferrum phosphoricum 6c   Indicated in febrile states and urinary tract involvement. Blood is bright red. Dose: every two hours for four doses.

China off. 6c   To control weakness associated with loss of blood. Helps to restore strength. Dose: every two hours for five doses.

Crotalus horridus 6c   Indicated in dark haemorrhages of fluid blood which does not clot easily, especially from intestines and rectum. Dose: three times daily for three days.

Sabina 6c   Indicated when the blood is bright red and, although fluid, clots immediately appear. Very useful in metrorrhagia. Dose: four times daily three hours apart.

Millefolium 6c   Indicated in haemorrhages of bright red blood associated with combined febrile symptoms. This is a useful remedy in haemoptysis and also when blood is prominent in the urine. Dose: every two hours for four doses.

Hamamelis 6c   Indicated in venous congestion with passive oozing haemorrhages. Dose: three times daily for two days.

Trillium pendulum 6c   This is associated with general weakness and dizziness after loss of blood, particularly from the uterus. Dose: every two hours for four doses.

3.   **Shock.**   Shock can result from injury or surgical interference and can lead to peripheral circulatory failure.

SYMPTOMS

The skin becomes cold and temperature falls to below normal. There is a fall in blood-pressure and a weak pulse rate together with shallow respirations. Severe shock can lead to coma.

TREATMENT

Arnica 30c   This remedy should be given in all cases. Dose: two doses usually suffice, two hours apart.

Bellis perennis 200c   This is a useful remedy to combat shock after surgical intervention. Dose: every three hours for three doses.

Carbo vegetabilis 6c   Indicated in cases of collapse and threatened coma. Body surface is cold. Dose: every two hours for
four doses.

Veratrum album 200c   Useful in surgical shock and indicated
when collapse is associated with cold perspiration. Dose: every
hour for four doses.

4. Oedema.   This is the term given to any abnormal amount
of fluid in tissue spaces. It can arise from various causes.

SYMPTOMS

Fluid swellings occur anywhere on the body surface and show
pitting on pressure. The swellings may arise from some inflammatory condition or be dependent on poor peripheral circulation
resulting from weak heart action. Oedema can also occur in body
cavities such as the pleural and pericardial sacs.

TREATMENT

Apis 6c   This is the main remedy for oedematous states whether
active from inflammation or passive as in chronic affections
of pleura and weak heart action. Dose: three times daily for
three days.

Antimonium tartaricum 30c   Indicated when oedema affects
the lung tissue, associated with great increase of mucus. Dose:
every two hours for four doses.

Prunus spinosa 6c   Useful in anascara and dependent parts such
as feet and lower limbs. Dose: three times daily for three days.

Digitalis 6c   Indicated if weak heart action is present. Dose:
three times daily for five days.

There are many other heart remedies to be considered, but they
will be dealt with under diseases of the heart.

5. Anemia.   This is the technical term for a deficiency of red
blood cells or of haemoglobin.

SYMPTOMS

Anaemia is characterised by pallor of the mucous membranes
and a weak, thready pulse. Jaundice and haemoglobinuria may
occur. Weakness and lethargy are common.

TREATMENT

China off. 30c   A useful remedy when there is extreme weakness and when slow leakage of blood is suspected. Dose: every two hours for four doses.

Arsenicum alb. 200c   This is a good remedy in long standing cases or pernicious anaemia states. The animal is exhausted and restless. Thirst is prominent, for small quantities. Dose: three times daily for three days.

Trinitrotoluene 30c   This remedy is associated with jaundice and haemoglobinuria. Faintness and palpitation are common symptoms. The urine is highly coloured. Dose: three times daily for five days.

Natrum muriaticum 1M   Indicated in long standing cases depending on deficient salt metabolism. Dose: night and morning for five days.

Silicea 1M   When there is an increase in the number of white cells leading to interference in haemoglobin function, this is a very useful remedy. Dose: twice weekly for four weeks.

VIII Diseases of Blood Vessels

1. **Arteritis.** This form of inflammation is common in horses infested with strongyle worms. It can lead to pathological changes in arteries such as the anterior mesenteric and the iliac, the former, when it occurs, giving rise to intermittent bouts of colic, and the latter to iliac thrombosis. Parasitic arteritis results in thickening of the artery walls due to inflammation. This can lead to the formation of a thrombus which in turn can lead to occlusion of the vessel. This is commonest in the anterior mesenteric artery. A specific form of arteritis also occurs and will be dealt with in the section on viral diseases.

TREATMENT

Calcarea fluorica 30c   Useful in removing fibrinoid deposits on the endothelium of the artery. Dose: three times daily for three days.

Kali hydriodicum 200c   Haemorrhagic infiltration of skin. Dose: three times daily for five days.

Note:—   In all cases of arteritis affecting mesenteric and iliac arteries, attention should be paid to removal of strongyle worms.

2. **Verminous aneurism.** This is of common occurrence in the horse and can interfere with intestinal blood supply.

SYMPTOMS

Recurrent attacks of colic take place and if the aneurism becomes infected with pyogenic bacteria, temperature rise occurs. Signs of peritonitis such as hardening of the abdominal wall may arise.

TREATMENT

Accessory homoeopathic treatment after worming includes consideration of the following remedies:-

Veratum viride 200c   Weak, intermittent pulse. There may be muscular twitchings and congestion of lungs. The animal is thirsty and the skin shows patches of sweating. Urine scanty. Dose: night and morning for four days.

Lycopodium 200c   Palpitation in thin subjects showing predisposition to liver disorders. Dose: three times daily for four doses.

Calcarea fluorica 30c   Glandular swellings with increased heart action. There may be an associated valvular incompetence. Dose: night and morning for four days.

3.   Venous Thrombosis.   This may arise as a sequel to strangles, and can affect large veins such as jugular or posterior vena cava.

SYMPTOMS

Pain on pressure over vein, engorgement and local oedema. The jugular vein, when affected, may stand out as a thickened cord-like structure.

TREATMENT

Vipera 30c   Associated jaundice and enlargement of liver. Dose: three times daily for five days.

Hamamelis 200c   Associated blood-shot involvement of eyes. Epistaxis is common and the veins of the throat become engorged. Dose: night and morning for four days.

IX Diseases of Lymphatic System

1. **Lymphangitis.**   This term implies inflammation of the lymphatic vessels of the legs, more particularly the hind legs. It is commonly associated with rest on full rations after a period of exercise.

SYMPTOMS
Initial shivering is followed by signs of febrile involvement, viz. rapid pulse and breathing, with hot dry mouth. The affected leg is raised from the ground and the animal shows signs of pain or discomfort, looking round at the affected limb. Heat, swelling and tenderness are present in the leg. A painful cord-like swelling develops on the inside of the limb, developing along the course of the lymphatic vessels. The swelling starts first in the groin and extends down the leg towards the fetlock. The early swelling pits on pressure indicating oedema. Severe cases are accompanied by the expression of a honey-coloured fluid on the surface of the skin.

TREATMENT
Aconitum napellus 6x   Should always be given in the early febrile stage. Dose: every hour for four doses.
Kali bichromicum 200c   Indicated when a viscid, honey-coloured discharge appears. Dose: three times daily for four days.
Calcarea fluorica 30c Useful in controlling involvement of associated lymph glands. Blood vessels are usually dilated. Dose: three times daily for four days.
Apis 6c   Indicated in the acute stage when oedematous swellings are prominent. Dose: three hourly for four doses.
Belladonna 200c   Useful when associated lymph glands are swollen and tender. Febrile signs are accompanied by dilation of pupils and a hot smooth skin. Dose: three hourly for four doses.

Lachesis 6c   This remedy may be needed if septic lymphangitis occurs, the underlying tissues showing cellulitis and the skin becoming dark bluish. Associated blood vessels are dilated and blood may ooze from rectum, being dark and fluid. Dose: three times daily for two days.

Rhus toxicodendron 1M   Associated with swelling and tenderness along the course of the lymphatic vessels, together with stiffness of the limb. The symptoms improve on exercise after rest. There may be an accompanying cellulitis. Dose: night and morning for four days.

2.   **Lymphadenitis.**   Inflammation of lymph glands may accompany bacterial infection or be associated with a neighbouring lymphangitis.

SYMPTOMS

Acute inflammation produces heat and swelling. Signs of pain are variable. Oedema accompanies lymphadenitis in the horse as a sequel to lymphangitis.

TREATMENT

Aconitum napellus 6c   Should be given as soon as possible in the early inflammatory stage. Dose: every hour for four doses.

Belladonna 1M   Indicated in acute cases when the glands are hot and tender. The animal shows excitement and dilated pupils. The pulse is full and bounding and the skin is hot and smooth. Dose: every two hours for four doses.

Phytolacca 30c   A good general remedy for swelling of glands. If the submaxillary glands are affected, the swelling extends to the neighbouring parotid salivary glands. This remedy is of benefit in both acute and chronic cases. Dose: night and morning for three days.

Kali hydriodicum 30c   A useful remedy when there is an associated local oedema. Coryza and lachrymation may be present. Dose: night and morning for five days.

Apis 6c   Indicated in acute cases when oedema of the gland substance is suspected. Fluid swellings surround the affected parts. Dose: every two hours for four doses.

Mercurius iod rub 6c   Especially suited for involvement of submaxillary glands which are enlarged and painful, especially on the left side. Dose: three times daily for three days.

Cistus 6c   A useful remedy in chronic lymphadenitis. The glands are indurated. The animal feels the cold and should be protected with a blanket. Throat glands may show a chronic suppuration. Dose: night and morning for one week.

Dulcamara 30c   Indicated when swelling and hardness of glands arise after exposure to cold and damp. Dose: night and morning for four days.

Hepar sulphuris 200c   This is a suitable remedy when suppuration of glands follows pyogenic infections. The animal is sensitive to cold and the glands are extremely tender and painful. Dose: night and morning for five days.

Silicea 1M   A good remedy for chronic involvement. Glands are hard and may contain inspissated pus. Dose: daily for one week.

3.   **Angioneurotic Oedema.**   This is the term used to denote oedema suddenly appearing, due to allergy and is usually of short duration. It is common in horses at pasture when flowers are in bloom. Affected animals commonly show recurrence after a previous attack.

SYMPTOMS
The head region is mostly affected, but lesions are frequently seen in the perineal region also. The eyes may become puffy and swollen along with similar involvement of the muzzle and cheeks. Lachrymation occurs along with salivation and occasionally rhinitis. Vulval swelling occurs in the mare when the perineal area is attacked.

TREATMENT
Apis 6c   This is a most useful remedy for oedematous swellings appearing especially round the eyes. Dose: every three hours for four doses.

Hypericum 1M   Indicated in cases associated with subcutaneous itching and a tendency to photosensitisation. Dose: every three hours for four doses.

Urtica urens 6c   Should be considered when the swellings are hot and itchy and there is general urticaria-like involvement over the body. Dose: every three hours for four doses.

Vespa 30c   Should be remembered as a possibly useful remedy when the condition is more confined to the face and eyes.

Throat and mouth severely swollen. Dose: every three hours for four doses.

Phosphorus 200c   Useful when the oedematous swellings are infiltrated with blood as a result of purpura-like haemorrhages. Dose: three times daily for two days.

Antipyrine 6c   Associated with intense pruritis and urticaria. Dose: three times daily for three days.

4.   Subcutaneous Haemorrhage.   This is sometimes seen in horses which have been upset by eating mouldy sweet clover hay, leading to capillary damage. This is known as dicoumerol poisoning.

SYMPTOMS

The main sign is a soft swelling with no skin involvement. It is usually painless.

TREATMENT

Melilotus 6x   Associated with general haemorrhage tendency: profuse epistaxis. Impaction of bowels occurs also. Dose: three times daily for four days.

Phosphorus 200c   Indicated when capillary damage leads to purpura-like haemorrhages and multiple small swellings. Dose: three times daily for two days.

Millefolium 6c   Haemorrhages of bright red blood occur from body orifices. Febrile symptoms are common with sustained high temperature. Dose: three times daily for three days.

Ficus religiosa 6c   Indicated in a general haemorrhage diathesis when there are accompanying respiratory symptoms, with vomiting of blood when coughing. Dose: every two hours for four doses.

Ipecacuanha 6c   A useful anti-haemorrhagic remedy when digestive upsets are present such as indigestion and slimy frequent stools. Dose: three times per day for three days.

Crotalus horridus 6c   Associated with decomposition of blood and generalised haemorrhages of dark, fluid non-coagulable blood. Septic involvement of lesions is common. Dose: every three hours for four doses.

Lachesis 30c   Indicated when cellulitis is associated with purpura-like haemorrhages of dark blood. Sometimes there is throat swelling. Dose: three times daily for three days.

Arnica 30c If the condition has arisen as a result of injury or multiple bruising. The skin over the haemorrhage swelling is discoloured. Dose: twice daily for one day.

Hamamelis 6c Indicated in general venous congestion. Throat vessels are engorged. Passive haemorrhages of dark blood. The haemorrhages under the skin are associated mainly with venous circulation. Dose: three times daily for three days.

Secale 30c Haemorrhages of dark, watery blood with a tendency to necrosis of tissue over the affected area. Epistaxis is common and the tongue is swollen making swallowing difficult. Dose: four times in one day.

X Diseases of Alimentary Canal

1. Stomatitis – Inflammation of Mouth.   This may arise from various causes, internal and external.

SYMPTOMS
The mouth shows redness. Pain and swelling are usually present. Febrile signs accompany the mouth inflammation. Ulceration of the buccal mucous membrane may occur, leaving a raw, red surface which may discharge purulent material, as a result of secondary infection.

TREATMENT
Aconitum napellus 6c   The early febrile stage. Dose: every hour for four doses.

Belladonna 200c   No salivation, but mouth red and shiny. pupils dilated and skin hot. Dose: every two hours for four doses.

Rhus toxicodendron 1M   Redness of tongue, with formation of small vesicles. Dose: every two hours for four doses.

Mercurius sol. 30c   Profuse ropy salivation, with discharge of purulent material. Dose: three times per day for two days.

Nitric acid 200c   Ulceration of the buccal mucous membrane occurs, leaving a raw surface. Dose: three times daily for two days.

Borax 6c   Vesicular involvement. This remedy very useful when the animal is afraid to move forward or downwards. Dose: three times daily for two days.

Lachesis 200c   Pronounced throat swelling, leading to difficulty in breathing and possible epistaxis. Dose: every hour for four doses.

Mercurius cyanatus 30c   Inflammation extends to the throat, with formation of whitish membrane. Dose: three times daily for three days.

Kali chloricum 6c   Signs of abdominal or hepatic disturbance. Dose: three times daily for three days.

2.   Paralysis of Lips.   This is usually seen as a result of injury or inflammation of nerves supplying the muscles of the lips.

SYMPTOMS
Lips appear flaccid and may hang loose, while saliva is not retained. Unable to pick food, or to drink water. If the condition is unilateral the lips are drawn away from the affected side.

TREATMENT
Gelsemium 200c   Condition arises as a result of toxaemia. Dose: three times daily for two days, followed by one dose every second day for three doses.
Arnica 10M   Paralysis results from an injury, one dose only, to be followed by other remedies according to indications.
Plumbum 30c   Signs of weakness or paralysis elsewhere. Dose: three times daily for three days.
Causticum 200c   Condition has origin in exposure to cold draughts. Dose: night and morning for three days.
Ammonium phos. 6c   Accompanying signs of tremulous or tottering gait. Dose: three times daily for three days.

3.   Ranula.   A cyst-like swelling under the tongue caused by obstruction to a salivary duct.

SYMPTOMS
A globular swelling appears under the tongue and may be unilateral or bilateral.

TREATMENT
Thuja 200c   Blisters on tongue, with inflammation of gums. Dose: three times daily for three days.
Apis 30c   Fluid in the ranula will be reduced by this remedy. Dose: three times daily for one week, followed by one dose daily of the same remedy in potency 200c for four doses.
Belladonna 1M   Inflammatory signs such as sensitivity to touch, with tenderness. Dose: every three hours for four doses.
Mercurius sol. 30c   Profuse salivation. Dose: three times daily for two days.

4.   Parotitis — Inflammation of Parotid Salivary Gland.   This may arise from exposure to cold and may also be a sequel to infectious diseases like strangles.

SYMPTOMS

Normally the gland on one side only is affected and becomes swollen, hard and painful. This hardness usually persists, but rarely becomes suppurative.

TREATMENT

Aconitum napellus 6c   Exposure to cold, producing an initial fever. This remedy should be used before giving any other. Dose: every hour for four doses.

Belladonna 1M   Gland initially hot and swollen. Signs of delirium may show. Dilated pupils, throbbing dull pulse. Dose: every hour for four doses.

Pulsatilla 6c   Right gland affected, with dry mouth and white coated tongue. Dose: three times daily for three days.

Calcarea fluorica 6c   Gland is of stony hardness. Inflammatory symptoms are reduced and associated lymph glands become involved. Dose: three times daily for three days.

Bryonia 6c   Origin is exposure to cold. Symptoms are relieved from pressure on the gland. Dose: three times daily for one day, followed by one dose night and morning of the potency 200c, for two days.

Baryta carb. 30c   This remedy is particularly useful for very young, or very old animals. Swelling extends to tonsils and throat veins may become prominent. Dose: three times daily for three days.

Ferrum phosphoricum 6c   A general hot feeling when the mouth is examined, with tonsillitis and ulceration of the throat. Dose: every two hours for four doses.

Kali bichromicum 30c   Tough, stringy discharge from mouth and throat. Soft palate may have membranous deposits. Pulse soft and slow. Dose: three times daily for three days.

Mercurius corrosivus 6c   Entire throat inflamed and swelling extends to lower neck. Inability to swallow. Salivation and slimy diarrhoea may accompany condition. Dose: three times daily for two days.

Phytolacca 30c   Throat bluish-red with swollen tonsils which may be dropsical. Membranous deposits on throat. Lachrymation may accompany throat symptoms. Dose: three times daily for three days.

Rhus toxicodendron 1M   Left gland usually affected. Small vesicles appear at corners of mouth. Tongue coated, red at edges. Throat red and inflamed. Redness and swelling of eyes, accompanied by orbital cellulitis. Dose: every two hours for four doses.

5.   Pharyngitis – Inflammation of Throat.   This condition may be dependent on change of weather or exposure to cold winds, or may be induced by change of food or work.

SYMPTOMS

Febrile symptoms first appear, accompanied by anorexia and difficulty in swallowing. The throat swells, becoming tender on pressure. Inflammation extends to the glands of the throat and under the ears. Respirations are increased and pulse is quickened.

TREATMENT

Aconitum napellus 6c   In early febrile stage, always use this remedy first. Dose: every hour for four doses.

Belladonna 200c   Full bounding pulse, dilated pupils. Tenderness and heat over throat glands. Hot, shiny skin. Animal usually excitable. Dose: every two hours for four doses.

Calcarea fluorica 6c   Glands under jaw and behind throat become stony hard. Dose: three times daily for three days.

Mercurius cyanatus 6c   Condition accompanied by membranous deposit on throat. Dose: three times daily for three days.

Rhus toxicodendron 1M   Vesicular involvement of mouth and tongue, with left-sided inflammation of throat glands. Dose: every two hours for four doses.

Bryonia 6c   Relief of symptoms on pressure over the throat, also when condition has arisen as result of exposure to cold dry winds. Dose: every two hours for four doses.

Alumen 6c   Tonsils enlarged and hardened. There may be general enlargement of superficial lymph glands on the body. Dose: three times daily for three days.

Aesculus hip. 30c   Veins of pharyngeal region swollen and distended. General abdomen discomfort. Liver dysfunction, signs of jaundice and pale stools. Dose: three times daily for two days, followed by one daily dose of potency 200c or 1M for four days.

Capsicum 6c   Inflammation extends backwards to base of ears. Useful remedy in less acute involvement. Dose: night and morning for four days.

6. Acute Indigestion.   Overeating or feeding on improper food accounts for this condition.

SYMPTOMS

These appear suddenly and include restlessness and signs of pain such as kicking at abdomen. Frequent rolling may accompany a tympanitic abdomen along with rising and lying down at short intervals. Sweating and increased pulse rate occur with discolouration of conjunctiva. The symptoms may abate and return just as badly after a short interval.

TREATMENT

Nux vomica 6c   Especially if condition arises from ingestion of indigestible fodder. Constipation usually present. Dose: every two hours for four doses.

Colchicum 6c   Tympanitic abdomen, animal passes flatus frequently. Dose: every two hours for three doses.

Colocynthis 6c   Animal rolls in acute pain, with head turned towards flank. Dose: every two hours for four doses.

Arsenicum alb. 1M   Animal restless, worse towards midnight, thirsty for small quantities of water. Skin dry and scurfy. Dose: every hour for three doses.

Abies canadensis 6c   Condition due to overeating. Flatulence prominent. Dose: every two hours for four doses.

Lobelia inflata 6c   Salivation and profuse sweating. Appetite often remains good. Flatulence often occurs. Dose: four times daily for one day.

Lycopodium 6c   Accompanying liver symptoms such as yellowish discolouration of conjunctiva and tenderness over liver region. Highly fermentable food aggravates. Dose: every two hours for four doses.

Carbo vegetabilis 6c   Abdomen tense due to flatulence, with comatose symptoms. Flatus very offensive. Symptoms worse lying down. Dose: every hour for four doses.

Nux moschata 6c   Excessive bloat. Difficulty passing a soft stool. Dose: every hour for four doses.

7. **Stomach Staggers.** In this condition, both stomach and nervous system are affected. It is more common in farm or heavy horses than in light breeds. It may arise if a horse gains access to corn after a period of fasting and then overeats.

SYMPTOMS
Constipation is present, dung being hard and shiny. Signs of colic appear and retention of urine is common. There may be passage of flatus and sweating is patchy in distribution. Mucous membranes of eye and mouth are tinged brick-coloured or yellowish. Symptoms of sleepiness and coma shortly appear and the animal may rest his head against any supporting object. The eyes are half-closed. Twitching of muscles may appear and the breathing is slow and laboured, while the pulse is full and hard. The eyesight becomes affected and hind-leg paralysis may supervene. These symptoms may progress to a more violent involvement of the nervous system, when the animal bangs his head against a wall, stamps the ground, rears up and may fall backwards. Dilated pupils and staring eyes are prominent, with hard, frequent pulse.

TREATMENT
Nux vomica 6c   Early stages of constipation. Dose: every two hours for four doses.
Opium 10M   Signs of sleepiness and coma, with bowels completely inactive. Dose: one dose only.
Conium 30c   Hind-leg paralysis tending to move forward. Dose: three times daily for three days, after which it may be necessary to follow with ascending potencies at regular intervals.
Belladonna 10M   Severe encephalitis, dilated pupils and full bounding pulse. Dose: every two hours for three doses.
Agaricus muscaris 200c   Head symptoms: falling over backwards, 'intoxication'. Dose: three times daily for three days.

8. **Loss of Appetite – Anorexia.**   Although not a disease, this can be troublesome and can affect a horse's performance and usefulness. It may be a symptom of concurrent disease and should be investigated in order to eliminate this possibility.

TREATMENT

In the absence of specific trouble, anorexia may be treated as follows:-

Nux vomica 6c   Condition dependent on weak digestion or full stomach. Dose: three times daily for three days.

Ornithogalum 1x   Signs of abdominal pain in stomach region, due to pyloric spasm or stenosis. Dose: every hour for four doses.

Vitamin B12 3x   This remedy frequently produces a return to appetite. Dose: three times daily for three days.

Anacardium 30c   Indefinite cases where more selected remedies have not produced result. Dose: three times daily for three days.

Arsenicum alb. 1M   Thirst for small sips of water. Dose: once daily for one week.

Hydrastis 6c   Catarrhal conditions such as coryza and muco-purulent lachrymation. The anorexia due to catarrhal gastritis. Dose: three times daily for three days.

China off. 30c   Bloated abdomen and general weakness. Bloating relieved by movement. Dose: every three hours for four doses.

9.   Constipation.   This condition accompanies many diseases, but may arise independently as a result of bad management, or allowing the animal access to rough forage. It may also be dependent on lack of sufficient fluid intake.

SYMPTOMS

Severe straining and passage of small hard lumps of dung, coated with slimy mucus. Spots of blood may be present on the lumps and in severe cases febrile signs may appear, such as reddened conjunctiva and quickened pulse.

TREATMENT

Nux vomica 6c   Uncomplicated cases, when there is ingestion of indigestible food. Dose: every two hours for three doses, in mild cases. In animals subject to a more chronic condition, give potency 1M night and morning for two days.

Sulphur 6c   Abdomen sensitive to pressure and colicky symptoms after drinking. This remedy can most usefully be employed in conjunction with Nux vom., giving the remedies in alternation.

Opium 1M Somnolence and lack of abdominal straining. Animal usually recumbent. Dose: every two hours for two doses.

Hydrastis 30c General catarrhal states. Signs of stiffness over lumbar region. Liver dysfunction and jaundice may be present. Dose: three times daily for three days.

Alumina 200c Bleeding from rectum. Severe straining, difficulty in passing urine. Dose: three times daily for three days.

Magnesia muriatica 6c Liver dysfunction, yellow tongue and other signs of jaundice may appear. Stools small and crumbly. Dose: three times daily for three days.

Collinsonia 6c Young animals with tendency to rectal prolapse, with possible anal irritation and flatulence. Dose: three times daily for four days.

Bryonia 6c Stools large, hard and may contain blood – especially in young animals. Dose: three times daily for three days.

Paraffinum 6c Straining, particularly in foals and young horses. Dose: three times daily for four days.

10.   Enteritis – Inflammation of Intestines.   This is a frequent occurrence and may be due to irritation from intestinal worms or to eating indigestible food. In acute cases, the inflammation may extend to the whole bowel.

SYMPTOMS

The condition usually arises slowly. Initial signs are restlessness, staring coat, dullness, rapid pulse and anorexia. Shivering may be present. Pain varies according to the severity of the condition. The abdomen is tucked up and is tender on pressure. There may be constipation, but when irritant materials have contributed to the cause, diarrhoea may be present. The conjunctiva becomes discoloured, while pulse is weak and thready. Prostration sets in as the condition advances, cold sweat appears and legs and ears become cold. Trembling and twitching also prominent symptoms in severe cases.

TREATMENT

Aconitum napellus 6c Early stages of febrile symptoms, animal anxious and restless. Dose: every hour for four doses.

Belladonna 1M Full bounding pulse, dilated pupils, hot shiny coat. Reddening of inside of nose and discolouration of cor junctiva. Dose: every two hours for four doses.

Mercurius corrosivus 30c   Thirst and salivation. Slimy motions streaked with blood, with cold sweaty perspiration. Dose: four times in one day, three hours apart.

Arsenicum alb. 1M   Restlessness, thirst for small quantities, weak thready pulse and symptoms worse after midnight. Coldness of legs and ears with watery motions, and cadaver-like odour. Dose: every two hours for four doses.

Colocynthis 6c   Symptoms of great pain. Animal lies down, head bent towards abdomen. Stools dysenteric and slimy, brought on by eating or drinking. Dose: four times daily, three hours apart, for two days.

Croton tiglium 30c   Severe diarrhoea results from inflammation of bowels. Stools watery and forcibly expelled. Dose: four times in one day only, three hours apart.

Sulphur 6c   Chronic cases. Mucous membrane of lips and mouth usually intensely red. Dose: three times daily for two days.

11. Dysentery.   Overwork or bad food can predispose to this condition. The acute form affects young animals particularly. Older animals may show a more chronic type.

SYMPTOMS

Anorexia, great thirst and small, rapid pulse. Respirations increased. Straining accompanied by signs of abdominal pain, such as kicking at abdomen. Motions are slimy and mucoid, containing whole blood. Fatty particles present.

TREATMENT

Aconitum napellus 6c   Early stages of feverish signs – quickened pulse and anxious expression. Dose: every hour for three doses.

Mercurius corrosivus 6c   Salivation   accompanies   condition. Worse at night. Dose: three times daily for two days.

Ipecacuanha 30c   Fatty particles in stool. Accompanying cough. Less straining than with Merc. Dose: three times daily for three days.

Arsenicum alb. 1M   Animal restless, motions watery and pale. Blood in the stool is diffused through the watery motion. Carrion-like odour from stool. Worse towards midnight, thirst for small quantities. Dose: every three hours for four doses.

Colocynth 6c   Severe colicky pains accompany restlessness and distension of abdomen. Animal lies down, bending head towards abdomen. Dose: every two hours for four doses.

Phosphoric acid 30c   Young animals show acute symptoms. Usually thin and may show skin irritation. Dose: every two hours for four doses.

Aloe 200c   Lumpy, jelly-like stools with rectal bleeding. Pain when passing stool. Much flatus present, with tenderness over liver region. Dose: three times daily for two days.

Cantharis 6c   Excessive tenesmus when passing stool. Shreds of mucus mixed with blood. Strangury, with small drops of bloody urine. Dose: every three hours for four doses.

Trombidium 30c   Pain before and after stool. Dysenteric motions after eating, stools thin, with straining. Dose: every two hours for three doses.

12. Diarrhoea – Superpurgation.   This may be an accompaniment of disease, or arise indefinitely as a result of improper feeding or change of diet.

SYMPTOMS

Frequently there is straining when passing evacuations and shreds of mucous membrane may be seen. Motions may be watery or mucoid, sometimes slimy, varying in colour according to the underlying cause. The stool may be passed with difficulty, shown by straining, or passively.

Superpurgation may arise from the overuse of purgatives or giving too large a dose. It may also be seen towards the end of febrile diseases, as a result of disordered metabolism e.g. liver dysfunction.

There is passage of flatus accompanied by signs of abdominal uneasiness e.g. looking round at flanks. If too much fluid is lost, the legs may get cold and the body temperature may fall.

TREATMENT

Mercurius corrosivus 200c   Motions slimy and may contain a little blood. The condition often worse during the night. Salivation. Dose: every two hours for four doses.

Arsenicum alb. 1M   Motions pale, watery and excoriate skin round anus. Signs of abdominal pain, thirst for small quantities of water. Worse after midnight, with restlessness and weakness. Odour from stools carrion-like. Dose: every two hours for four doses.

Bryonia 6c   Condition brought on by cold dry winds, or sudden change of temperature, or by drinking large quantities of cold water. Dose: three times daily for three days.

Nux vomica 6c   Overeating or partaking of indigestible food. Diarrhoea may be preceded by attacks of colic.

Dulcamara 200c   Attacks of dairrhoea follow exposure to damp. Stools green and slimy. More prevalent in summer, after sudden fall in temperature. Dose: every two hours for four doses.

Colocynth 6c   Attack is accompanied by severe abdominal pain. Animal lies down and rises frequently, bending neck towards abdomen. Food and drink produces jelly-like slimy stools. Dose: every half-hour for four doses, followed by one dose every four hours for two doses.

Croton tiglium 6c   Severe watery diarrhoea, with great expulsive movements, brought on even by small quantities of water. Dose: three times daily for two days.

China off. 30c   Weakness due to loss of body fluid. This remedy is especially useful in chronic cases. Dose: three times daily for three days.

Podophyllum 6c   Long-standing cases. Stools watery and foetid. Attacks worse in morning. There may be prolapse of rectum. Very useful in young animals. Dose: three times daily for three days.

13.   Colic.   This condition is referred to as spasmodic or flatulent, according to the symptoms arising. Spasmodic colic implies a cramping or spasm of the muscular coat of a portion of the large intestine. Animals of an excitable temperament are more disposed to the condition than those of a more lethargic nature. Flatulent colic, as the name implies, is accompanied by excessive formation of flatus. In each type the pulse becomes thready and the conjunctiva discoloured.

SYMPTOMS
Initially, there is restlessness, pawing the ground and kicking at the abdomen. The animal lies down and may roll violently, or it may lie flat, occasionally looking round at the flank. These spasms pass off but return after a short interval. The expression

is anxious and respirations are increased. With flatulent colic there are additional symptoms, tympany and tense abdomen. There are rumbling noises from the bowel and frequent passage of flatus.

TREATMENT

Aconitum napellus 6c   Always in the early stages, one dose every hour for four doses.

Belladonna 1M   Full bounding pulse early in condition, sweating, dilated pupils and excitability. Skin hot and smooth. Dose: every two hours for four doses.

Colchicum 6c   Distension of abdomen and rumbling of flatus. Lower parts of the bowel become distended and can be felt on right side. Animal tends to remain standing. Dose: every hour for three doses.

Colocynth 1M   When spasmodic colic has severe pain and appears to result from having eaten green food. Motions watery, with wind. Dose: every four hours for four doses.

Nux vomica 6c   If attack brought on by eating indigestible food or overeating. Straining to pass dung and urinate. Animal lies on his side looking uneasy, bending head towards flank. Dose: every two hours for four doses.

Ammonium causticum 6c   Preponderance of wind, respirations becomes laboured and short, with discharge of mucus from nostrils. Dose: every two hours for four doses.

Note:—   In extremely acute cases, it may be necessary to administer medicines every ten or fifteen minutes. Generally five or six doses should be sufficient, followed by the extended times outlined above.

XI Diseases of Liver

1. **Jaundice.** This occurs as a symptom of inflammation of the liver. Sluggish function without inflammation may also produce jaundice. It is sometimes also associated with pneumonia. Obstruction of the bile ducts is also an obvious cause.

SYMPTOMS

The mucous membranes of the eye, mouth and nose become tinged with yellow and skin also shows this discolouration. Urine becomes dark green, because of the presence of bile. Constipation may be present, faeces light in colour. Oedema of limbs may supervene.

TREATMENT

Berberis vulgaris 30c   Sluggish liver conditions with tenderness over lumbar region. Skin yellowish, urinary symptoms present. Dose: three times daily for three days.

Carduus marianus 6c   Inflammation of liver accompanied by tenderness over hepatic region. Jaundice produces golden-coloured urine. Dose: three times daily for three days.

Chelidonium 6c   Pain and tenderness over right shoulder area. Strong yellow discolouration of visible mucous membranes. Obstruction of bile ducts. Dose: three times daily for three days.

Chionanthus 6c   Jaundice produces yellow putty-like stools. Liver enlarged. Dose: one times daily for three days.

China off. 30c   Weakness and debility. Abdominal pain. Stools yellow and fluid, increasing weakness; Dose: every three hours for four doses.

Hydrastis 30c   Catarrahl state of bile ducts leading to a gleety condition of urine. Indigestion due to catarrhal gastritis. Pain and stiffness over back. Dose: three times daily for three days.

Lycopodium 200c   Flatulent state. Indifferent appetite. Abdominal tympany after eating. Mucous membranes greyish-yellow and urine loaded with red sediment. Dose: night and morning for five days.

Leptandra 6c Jaundice cases showing bowel haemorrhage, giving black, foul-smelling stools. Tongue thickly coated and yellow. Portal circulation becomes disturbed. Dose: three times daily for three days.

Magnesia muriatica 30c Enlargement of liver with difficulty in urination. Jaundice and abdominal pain pronounced. Dose: night and morning for four days.

2.   Hepatitis.   Inflammation of the liver parenchyma may be caused by a number of varying substances, some in horses being specific viral or other infectious agents. Acute and chronic forms are recognised.

SYMPTOMS

In the acute form, the animal is dull and disinclined to move. Muscular weakness and anorexia are common signs and there may be nervous excitability. Urine is scanty and high coloured. The faeces are clay-coloured and soft after initial constipation in the early anorexia stage. Yawning and lethargy are seen and there may be a tendency to fall forward or press the head against a wall or any convenient object. There is conjunctival discoloura-tion and the mucous membranes of the mouth and nose are yellow and furred-looking. Pain over the right scapular areas produces slight lameness and is also evident on palpation of the liver area. Photosensitisation may occur in animals which are exposed to sunlight and fed on green food.

Chronic states may show oedema and jaundice more commonly than in the acute form. Ecchymotic haemorrhages are frequently seen and there is more tendency to head pressing.

TREATMENT

Phosphorus 200c Acute form. Stools whitish, either soft or hard. Jaundice and purpura-like haemorrhages occur, urine shows haemoglobinuria and is muddy-looking. Pain in abdo-men. Dose: three times daily for three days.

Aloe 200c Abdominal fullness, excessive flatus. Urine scanty, high-coloured. Stools contain much clotted mucus and are very loose. Dose: night and morning for three days.

Bryonia 6c   Better at rest. Relief from pressure over liver. Dry coughing may accompany condition. Stools hard, dark, dry, urine scanty and hot. Dose: three times daily for three days.

Carduus marianus 6c   Both acute and chronic cases. Urine deep yellow, due to jaundice. Stools deep yellow, alternate between constipation and diarrhoea. Ascites common in chronic state. Dose: three times daily for two days in acute stage: night and morning for two weeks in the more chronic.

Chelidonium 6c   Acute stage, showing prominent jaundice, stiffness and pain over right scapular area. Dose: three times daily for three days.

Hydrastis 30c   Catarrhal hepatitis indicated by gleety mucus in the urine and evidence of catarrhal inflammations elsewhere, such as rhinitis and catarrhal cough. Dose: night and morning for five days.

Hepar sulphuris 200c   Suspected hepatic abscess, shown by presence of purulent material in urine, which has a greasy look. Suppurative involvement may be evident elsewhere, e.g. purulent rhinitis. Dose: night and morning for five days.

Lycopodium 200c   More chronic form, in the early stages of cirrhosis. Ascitis usually present. Urine contains reddish sediment, and is passed copiously during the night. Dose: night and morning for two weeks.

Mercurius dulcis 6c   Chronic hepatitis, with loose, slimy stools, frequently blood-stained. Colitis may be present. Dropsical states common. Dose: three times daily for one week.

XII Diseases of Kidney and Bladder

1. Glomerulo-nephritis.   Streptococcal infection may be a contributory cause of this condition in the horse.

SYMPTOMS
The main signs are oliguria and threatened anuria, while in the later stages uraemic signs appear, including increased respirations, sleepiness, intermittent diarrhoea and finally coma. The urine contains high protein together with albumen casts and erythrocytes. Chronic cases show a clear urine, with a low specific gravity and devoid of protein. The acute stage of glomerulo-nephritis is marked by swelling of the kidney substance together with tissue oedema. Pain and tenderness over the kidneys and loins is a fairly constant sign. Increased thirst may accompany the chronic form, owing to salt retention.

TREATMENT
Apis 6c   Renal oedema in the acute form. Urine shows albuminous casts. Dose: every two hours for four doses.

Arsenicum alb. 6c   Scanty urine showing high albumen content and drops of blood. The animal is restless and thirsty for small quantities. There is a harsh, dry coat. Symptoms worse after midnight. Dose: every two hours for four doses.

Belladonna 1M   Acute cases showing excitement and dilated pupils. Full bounding pulse and hot smooth skin. Straining to pass urine which is scanty and loaded with phosphates. Haematuria is common. Dose: every two hours for four doses.

Berberis vulgaris 30c   Marked tenderness over loins. Urine contains mucus and a reddish sandy sediment. Urination is frequent. Dose: every three hours for four doses.

Mercurius sol. 30c   Urine scanty, with greenish mucus sediment which may contain pus and blood. Urine is dark-coloured.

Dose: three times daily for four days.

Lycopodium 200c   Urine profuse during the night. Tendency to retention with thick reddish sediment. Dose: night and morning for five days.

Thlaspi bursa 6c   Frequent urination with haematuria and a tendency to sand and gravel. Urine heavy with phosphates. Dose: three times daily for two days.

Terebinthina 6c   Urine bloody and difficult to expel. Pronounced sweetish odour. Condition often associated with infections. Dose: three times daily for three days.

Phosphorus 200c   Acute cases showing blood in urine. Blood is diffused through urine, giving a brownish appearance. Dose: night and morning for three days.

Eucalyptus 6c   Suppurative involvements following infections. Urine contains pus. Dose: three times daily for five days.

Kali chloricum 6c   Associated jaundice and haemoglobinuria. Urine is albuminous, plentiful and high in phosphates. Dose: three times daily for three days.

Natrum muriaticum 200c   Chronic cases showing a pale urine of low specific gravity. There is usually salt retention leading to thirst and anaemia. Dose: night and morning for one week.

2.   Nephrosis.   This term includes degenerative and inflammatory lesions of the renal tubules. It constitutes a chronic illness characterised by polyuria, emaciation and dehydration. It is frequently associated with toxaemia.

SYMPTOMS

In the acute stage diminution of urine occurs with increased protein in the urine. Chronic cases show polyuria, but degenerative changes in the glomerule sometimes produce a stage of oliguria. The chronic stage is also marked by urine of a low specific gravity.

TREATMENT

Aconitum napellus 6c   Acute stage, urine scanty and reddish. Dose: hourly for four doses.

Arsenicum alb. 200c   Urine hot and excoriating. There may be carrion-like diarrhoea. Urine contains casts. Symptoms worse after midnight. Dose: two hourly for four doses.

Acetic acid 6c   Chronic cases showing polyuria and pale urine.

There may be an accompanying ascites. Dose: three times daily for four days.

Aesculus hip. 30c Associated hepatic cases. Urine scanty and dark. Pain over left lumbar region. Dose: three times daily for four days.

Berberis vulgaris 30c Sacral and lumbar pains. Polyuria alternates with oliguria. Dose: night and morning for five days.

Argentum nitricum 30c Turbidity of urine with sweet smell. Frequent passage of urine and incoordination of movement. Dose: night and morning for four days.

Natrum muriaticum 200c Emaciation, thirst and anaemia in chronic cases. Dose: night and morning for one week.

Cantharis 30c Acute inflammatory stage showing severe straining and passage of bloody urine, which contains shreds of mucous membrane. Dose: two hourly for four doses.

Plumbum 30c Frequent straining and signs of abdominal pain. Urine scanty and expelled drop by drop. Dose: night and morning for one week.

Conium 200c Old animals showing weakness of hind limbs. Nervous weakness. Inability to expel urine properly. Dose: night and morning for five days.

Note:— General signs of nephritis include a characteristic stance of the animal in the acute stage. The hind legs become stiff and straddled and there is disinclination to move. The loins are arched and hot and tender to the touch. Thirst is evident and the urine, which may contain blood, is passed with difficulty and in small amounts. The pulse is hard and quick.

3. Diabetes Insipidus – Profuse Staling. In this condition there is excessive passage of urine. It may be caused by damaged food, e.g. mouldy hay or oats.

SYMPTOMS
Appetite is diminished and the animal tires easily. Sweating is common. Thirst is prominent and the urine becomes profuse and clear.

TREATMENT
Phosphoric acid 6c Polyuria worse during the night. Urine contains phosphates and has a milky appearance. Dose: three

times daily for five days.

Acetic acid 6c   Excessive thirst and debility. Abdominal symptoms such as ascites are common. Dose: three times daily for five days.

Alfalfa 1x   Increase in the amount of urea and phosphates in the urine. Frequency of urination accompanying the polyuria. Dose: four times daily for three days.

Uranium nitricum 6c   Increase of sugar in the urine, plus increased flow. Accompanying emaciation with tendency to dropsy. Dose: three times daily for five days.

Argentum metallicum 30c   Urine may be turbid, has sweetish odour. Dose: night and morning for three days.

Eupatorium purpureum 6c   Strangury at beginning of urination. Urine appears milky and may contain blood. Dose: three times daily for two days.

Helonias 6c   Urine is albuminous, profuse and clear. This remedy is especially indicated in mares and fillies. Dose: three times daily for four days.

Sinapis nigra 6c   Frequent urging, flow copious. Dose: four times daily for one day.

4.   Haematuria.   Blood in urine may be associated with injuries or toxaemia from a systemic disease. It may be seen in mares after foaling.

SYMPTOMS

When due to injuries, the loins are hot and the condition tends to recur. When due to toxaemia, the usual febrile signs are present e.g. increased pulse and respiration.

TREATMENT

Aconitum napellus 6c   Early febrile stage of toxaemic state. Animal tense and anxious. Dose: every hour for four doses.

Arnica 30c   Condition due to injuries, urine shows dark brown sediment. Dose: night and morning for two days.

Terebinthina 200c   Urine has sweetish odour. Strangury common, with tendency to suppression. Useful remedy in toxaemic states. Dose: night and morning for four days.

Belladonna 200c   In haematuria, where there is no history of injuries or systemic affections. Passage of urine frequent, with signs of excitement. Dose: every three hours for four doses.

Coccus cacti 6c   Great difficulty passing urine. Red sediment containing calculi and urates. Dose: four times in twenty-four hours.

Crotalus horridus 6c   Urine dark and albuminous, containing casts. Associated with dark haemorrhages elsewhere. Dose: three times daily for three days.

Hamamelis 6c   Increased urination, with venous congestion and passive haemorrhages. Dose: night and morning for five days.

Millefolium 6c   When bright red blood in urine is associated with similar haemorrhages elsewhere. Dose: three times daily for three days.

Nitric acid 6c   Urine contains albumen and smells strongly of ammonia. Cloudy phosphatic urine may alternate with clear urine in old animals. Dose: three times daily for three days.

Pareira brava 6c   Thick urine containing much mucus, with great straining and signs of general pain. Dose: three times daily for three days.

Phosphorus 200c   Acute febrile state, with signs of liver disturbance, e.g. jaundice and haemoglobinuria. Purpura-like haemorrhages may be seen on visible muccous membranes. Dose: night and morning for three days.

Uva ursi 6c   Great accumulation of clotted blood and mucus in the urine, which may be bile stained and contain pus. Dose: three times daily for three days.

5.   Cystitis.   Inflammation of the bladder can arise from an extension of infection from some part of the urogenital tract. It may also arise as a sequel to calculus formation.

SYMPTOMS
There is general constitutional involvement; pulse and respiration are increased. There is trembling of the hind legs, accompanied by frequent straining to pass urine which may be so scanty as to pass drop by drop. Urine is blood-stained and contains mucus and sabulous material. Paralysis of the muscular coat of the bladder is common in chronic cases, shown by an inability to retain urine.

TREATMENT
Aconitum napellus 6c   In the early febrile involvement when

pulse and respiration are increased. Dose: every hour for four doses.

Cantharis 30c   Much straining and scanty amounts of bloody urine. There is hyperexcitability and signs of sexual irritability. Dose: night and morning in chronic cases, for one week. In acute cases, give one dose every hour for four doses.

Thlaspi bursa 6c   Chronic cystitis, when urine contains brick-coloured sediment of gravelly material. Dose: three times daily for one week.

Copaiva 6c   Catarrhal cystitis, shown by increase of mucus in the urine. Pain over the bladder area and urine has a sweetish smell. Dose: three times daily for three days.

Nux vomica 30c   When ineffectual urging is associated with digestive upsets. Dose: three times daily for two days.

Camphor 6c   Strangury, associated with a general collapsed state. Pulse slow, body icy cold. Dose: every hour for four doses.

Cubebs 6c   Frequent urination and catarrhal inflammation of the urogential tract. A great amount of mucus in the urine. Dose: three times daily for three days.

Dulcamara 30c   Catarrhal cystitis resulting from exposure to cold or damp. Urine contains a thick mucus or purulent sediment. Dose: three times daily for three days.

Eucalyptus 6c   Catarrhal inflammation, while urine contains blood and pus. Urination profuse. Dose: four times daily, three hours apart, for one day.

Eupatorium purpureum 6c   Animal shows uneasiness on passage of urine, which may be profuse and milky. Dose: three times daily for three days.

Oleum santali 1x   Chronic state. Urine shows thick catarrhal deposit. Dose: three times daily for one week.

Uva ursi 6c   Chronic state, where urine is slimy and accompanied by pain and tenesmus. Dose: three times daily for one week.

Sabina 6c   Bright blood in urine. Pain over kidneys and bladder. This remedy may act better in mares or fillies, especially when there are uterine symptoms in the former. Dose: night and morning for one week.

6.   Embolic Nephritis.   This condition has been reported in foals as a sequel to infection by Shigella species.

SYMPTOMS

The urine contains blood and pus. Pain and tenderness over the kidney area accompanied by abdominal discomfort.

TREATMENT

Hepar sulphuris 200c Animal shows extreme sensitivity to pressure or to cold draughts. Dose: night and morning for five days.

Silicea 30c Excessive sweating, but symptoms less acute than those calling for Hepar sulph. Pus is thin and greyish. Dose: night and morning for six days.

7. **Pyelonephritis.** This usually arises from ascending infection of the urinary tract.

SYMPTOMS

Presence of pus in the urine. This may arise from infection of the kidney pelvis, from a suppurative nephritis or from cystitis and urethritis.

TREATMENT

Hepar sulphuris 200c There is frequently an accompanying suppurative lymphadenitis. Pain and swelling over the loins. Excessive reaction to cold winds or draughts or to touch on kidney area. Dose: night and morning for four days.

Silicea 30c More chronic case. Pus in urine is creamy-white. Dose: night and morning for one week.

Streptococcus nosode 30c A useful supplementary remedy to be given along with other indicated medicines. Dose: once daily for three days.

Mercurius corrosivus 200c Urine is slimy and contains whole blood and greenish pus. Dose: night and morning for four days.

Benzoic acid 6c When condition results from a primary catarrhal or suppurative cystitis. Urine strong-smelling with high uric acid content. Dose: three times daily for three days.

Kali bichromicum 200c General catarrhal inflammation of mucous membranes, especially respiratory. Urine contains albumen and casts and is excessively mucous in character. Dose: night and morning for five days.

Uva ursi 6c Slimy urine, with tendency to calculus formation.

Often with urticaria and respiratory symptoms such as dyspnoea. Mucus and pus in urine has a sticky, colloidal character showing as large clots. Dose: three times daily for five days.

Epigea 1x   When chronic cystitis leads to a secondary pyelonephritis. Urine contains fine gravel deposit, with pus and haemoglobinuria. Dose: three times daily for five days.

Populus tremuloides 1x   Asscompanying gastric symptoms, especially in the older animal, and particularly in pregnant mares. Dose: three times daily for five days.

8.   Urolithiasis.   This condition may arise from stasis of urine. various factors contribute, but frequently the origin lies in sluggish liver function.

SYMPTOMS

Obvious difficulty in passing urine, which is scanty and bloodstained. Signs of pain include kicking at belly and looking round at the flanks. The penis is usually relaxed during attempts to urinate.

TREATMENT

Thlaspi bursa 30c   Condition due to chronic cystitis. Blood in urine with brick-coloured sediment. Dose: night and morning for one week.

Lycopodium 200c   Hepatic symptoms, with blood-stained urine containing red sediment — the early stages of calculus formation. Dose: night and morning for seven days.

Berberis vulgaris 30c   Associated with liver dysfunction. Tenderness over loins and uric acid deposits in the urine, which also contains mucus. Dose: night and morning for five days.

Sarsaparilla 6c   Pain at the beginning and at the end of urination, especially at the end. Urine contains gravelly deposit and is slimy. Dose: three times daily for three days.

Coccus cacti 6c   Dark urine containing whole blood and urates. Small calculi may be present. Considerable urging and tenesmus. Dose: three times daily for five days.

Solidago 6c   When urine is slimy and has thick sediment, but has a clear colour and offensive smell. Dose: three times daily for four days.

Ocimum ganum 30c   Cases which show a uric acid diathesis.

Long crystals of uric acid may appear in urine, which has a characteristic heavy smell. Urine thick and purulent. Dose: night and morning for five days.

9.   Paralysis of the Bladder.   In the early stages of paralysis, the bladder remains full and dribbling of urine takes place. The bladder wall loses its muscle tone and the result is a build up to a chronic cystitis.

TREATMENT

Gelsemium 200c   There is a profuse flow of pale urine which is expelled passively when the bladder becomes full. Dose: night and morning for five days.

Conium 30c   When passage of urine starts and stops frequently. There is difficulty in expulsion. Condition may be accompanied by weakness of back and hind limbs, shown by difficulty in rising. Dose: three times daily for four days.

XIII Affections of the Skin

1. Pityriasis or Dandruff. The term implies an accumulation of bran-like scales on the skin. It has various causes, such as dietary, parasitic, fungoid, etc.

SYMPTONS
There is an accumulation of scales on the skin, unaccompanied by itching. The scales are more prominent where there is long hair, e.g. under the mane. The coat is dry and harsh.

TREATMENT
Arsenicum alb. 1M   This is especially adapted to fine-skinned animals. The temperament is usually restless and there is thirst for small quantities. Dose: once daily for two weeks.
Kali sulphuricum 6c   Indicated where there are accompanying symptoms of gastric and respiratory upset. There may be an associated eczema showing papular eruption. Dose: three times daily for three days.
Lycopodium 200c   Thickening of the skin which later becomes dry and shrunken. Dose: night and morning for one week.
Natrum muriaticum 200c   When condition is associated with a greasy skin. There may be increased passage of urine with a low specific gravity. Dose: night and morning for one week.
Graphites 6c   Skin rough and hard, showing a streaky discharge. Dose: three times daily for one week.
Sulphur 6c   Skin generally unhealthy-looking and dirty. There may be a musty smell. Folds of skin tend to become excoriated. Dose: three times daily for one week.

2. Parakeratosis. This is a condition where keratinisation of epithelial cells is incomplete.

SYMPTOMS

The condition shows as a lesion often confined to the flexor aspects of the joints. It is shown first as reddening, followed by thickening of the skin. A greyish discolouration becomes super-imposed. Fissuring takes place and a raw red surface remains.

TREATMENT

Kali arsenicum 30c   Lesions worse under warm conditions. There may be an associated itching. Dose: night and morning for one week.

Cantharis 200c   Acute state, showing itching and reddening of skin. Straining at urination probable, urine being passed drop by drop. Dose: night and morning for four days.

Graphites 6c   Persistent dryness of skin with, or without, exudation. Dose: three times daily for four days.

Sulphur iodatum 6c   Accompanying papular eruption, usually with reddening and itching. Dose: night and morning for one week.

3. Impetigo.   This condition is characterised by the appearance of small vesicles surrounded by an erythematous zone. It is usually staphylococcal in origin, and found frequently on the hairless parts of the body.

SYMPTOMS

The vesicles at first contain a clear fluid, but later become pustular and then go on to scale formation. They remain separate as a rule. Secondary infection after rupture of the pustule can lead to pyogenic involvement.

TREATMENT

Antimonium tartaricum 6c   Vesicles and pustules are surrounded by a bluish red mark. There may be an accompanying respiratory distress. Debility and sweating are prominent symptoms. Dose: three times daily for three days followed by one dose daily for four days.

Mezereum 30c   Condition associated with stiffness and involvement of bones. Intense itching of vesicles which have a reddish surround. Dose: night and morning for five days.

Cantharis 200c   Vesicles intensely itching and burning, together with accompanying strangury, the urine being blood-stained and passed drop by drop. Dose: three times daily for two days followed by one dose daily for three days.

Rhus venenata 30c   Underlying skin dark red. Itching and erysipeloid inflammation. Dose: night and morning for four days.

Hepar sulphuris 200c   Secondary infection leads to the formation of purulent small ulcers. Dose: night and morning for five days.

4.   Urticaria.   This is an allergic condition characterised by wheals or raised oedematous plaques on the skin. They appear quickly and are usually multiple.

SYMPTOMS

The plaques are tender to the touch. If dependent on insect bites or stings, itching may be present, but otherwise this is absent. Diarrhoea is usually present.

TREATMENT

Antimonium crudun 6c   Much itching and plaques are small and numerous. Dose: three hourly for four doses.

Apis 6c   Plaques hot and tender and contain fluid and are usually large. Dose: two hourly for four doses. Abdomen mainly affected, with tendency for the condition to become chronic. Dose: three times daily for four days.

Antipyrene 6c   Condition accompanied by angio-neurotic oedema, which appears very suddenly. Dose: two hourly for four doses.

Fragaria 6c   Accompanying erysipelatous inflammation, with an associated body swelling. Dose: three hourly for four doses.

Astacus fluv. 30c   Liver complaints, e.g. jaundice accompany the condition. Cervical lymph glands swollen. Dose: three times daily for three days.

Natrum muriaticum 200c   Accompanying alopecia and passage of large quantities of pale urine. Dose: once daily for ten days.

Urtica Urens 6c   Plaques hot and itchy, with a tendency to oedema. Urine usually contains uric acid deposits. Dose: three times daily for three days.

5.   Eczema.   This term covers skin complaints which produce an inflammation of epidermal cells. It can arise from internal or external factors. It may be environmental in origin, or be dependent on excessive sweating or repeated wetting.

SYMPTOMS
The initial lesion is erythematous, followed by weeping of the skin. Itching is usually intense and alopecia may occur.

TREATMENT
Sulphur 30c   Lesion red and looks wet. Itching intense, worse from warmth. Dose; night and morning for five days.

Arsenicum alb 1M   Dry eczema. Animal is thirsty and seeks warmth. Symptoms worse after midnight, animal becoming more restless. Dose: once daily for two weeks.

Rhus toxicodendron 1M   Condition is vesicular and itchy. Stiffness is relieved by movement. Dose: once daily for five days.

Bovista 6c   Pimply eruption with crust formation and abnormal pain. Dose: three times daily for four days.

Antimonium crudum 6c   Eczema accompanied by stomach upsets. Worse at night. Dose: night and morning for three days.

Anacardium 200c   Nervousness. Skin reddish and very itchy, with vesicular eruption. Dose: night and morning for five days.

Petroleum 200c   Blistery eruptions with tendency to suppuration of cracked skin, which bleeds easily. Skin usually dry. Dose: night and morning for one week.

Psorinum 30c   Dry, lustreless skin with severe pruritis. The associated lymph glands are swollen. Sometimes an oily skin has ulceration which heals slowly. An unpleasant smell accompanies the eczema. Dose: night and morning for one week.

Graphites 6c   Discharge of sticky, honey-coloured fluid. Dose: three times daily for three days.

Cantharis 200c   Severe vesicular eczema. Strangury and blood-stained urine. Dose: night and morning for five days.

Kali Arsenicum 30c   Severe pruritis in chronic states. Worse from a change of weather. Lesion dry and scaly. Dose: night and morning for ten days.

6.   Dermatitis.   This term implies an inflammation of the true skin — the dermis — and the epidermis. It may be bacterial, mycotic or viral in origin and an allergic form is common in the horse.

SYMPTOMS

Erythema is the first sign. Vesicular lessions may then occur, followed by oedema of the subcutaneous tissues in severe cases, leading to cellulitis if the condition persists. Shock may be present in the early stages and toxaemia may occur.

TREAMENT

Arsenicum alb. 1M   Dry dermatitis. Thirsty, restless and worse after midnight. Dose: one dose per day for ten days.

Rhus toxicodendron 1M   Vesicles may form in the early erythematous stage. Stiffness of joints. Dose: one dose three times daily for two days.

Antimonium tartaricum 30c   Early stages of vesicular formation. Respiratory symptoms sometimes accompany this condition. Dose: one dose night and morning for three days.

Arnica 30c   Shock symptoms in the early stages. Dose: one dose six hourly for two doses.

Aconitum napellus 6c   Febrile symptoms and toxaemia. Dose: one dose two hourly for four doses.

Thuja 200c   Chronic state, showing thickening of the skin. Dose: one dose per day for two weeks.

7.   Photosensitisation.   This condition in which the unpigmented parts of the skin show sensitivity to sunlight is sometimes seen in piebald or skewbald animals. It is a sensitisation of the superficial layers of the skin to light and may lead to dermatitis.

SYMPTOMS

Lesions are restricted to unpigmented areas and may accompany liver disturbance such as jaundice. The lesions are always confined to the upper part of the body. The early signs may be erythema and oedema.

TREATMENT

Hypericum 1M   Accompanying pruritis. Dose: three hourly for four doses.

Chelidonium 1M   Signs of jaundice, pain and stiffness over the right shoulder area. Dose: once daily for one week.

Rhus venenata 30c   Dermatitis and blister formation. Dose: night and morning for four days.

Antimonium crudum 6c   Skin dry and itchy, with tendency to scab formation. Dose: night and morning for five days.

8.   Alopecia.   Loss of hair may be due to metabolic or dietetic errors. The skin may appear shiny and thinner than usual.

TREATMENT

Lycopodium 200c   Frequent skin ulceration together with gastric and hepatic disorders. Dose: night and morning for one week.

Pix liquida 6c   Skin irritation accompanied by respiratory disorder. Dose: night and morning for five days.

Calcarea fluorica 6c   Helpful in skin conditions which heal slowly, e.g. ulcers and fissures. Dose: three times daily for three days.

Thyroidinum 200c   In generalised alopecia when it is suspected that the thyroid gland is at fault. Dose: once daily for two weeks.

Note:—   It may be necessary to continue treatment on a higher potency and for a longer period, if there is only partial improvement with any of the above remedies.

9.   Seborrhoea.   This is excessive secretion of sebum on the skin. In horses one of the main types is greasy heel starting as a dermatitis or eczema and leading to secondary infection. Greasy heel is commonest in the hind feet of horses accustomed to standing for long periods in damp, unhygenic stables.

SYMPTOMS

The skin becomes thick and greasy and small vesicles appear. In cases of greasy heel, lameness appears first, followed by pain due to abrasions on the skin which may extend down to the coronary band.

TREATMENT

Arsenicum alb. 1M   Use in the early stages before secretion of sebum becomes profuse. Dose: once daily for one week.

Graphites 6c   Secretion is sticky and honey-coloured, skin generally rough and dry. Eczematous lesions appear in the fissures of the skin and bends of the joints. Dose: three times daily for five days.

Antimonium crudum 30c   Vesicles appear, accompanying thickening of the skin. Dose: night and morning for one week.

Thuja 200c   A most valuable remedy in greasy heel. Dose: once daily for ten days.

Note:−   Externally an application of *Arsenicum* Lotion is useful. Other applications such as *Sulphuric acid* and *Thuja* lotions may be used.

10.   Hyperkeratosis.   In this condition keratinised cells accumulate on the skin surface.

SYMPTOMS

Skin becomes corrugated and hairless. Excessive thickening occurs accompanied by dryness and scale formation. Fissuring occurs and may lead to secondary infection.

TREATMENT

Arsenicum alb. 1M   Useful when continued over several weeks with intervals between treatments. Dose: once daily for one week, followed by several weeks of no treatment. If, during the interval, improvement has been noted, but ceases, it is then advisable to continue with this remedy in a higher potency, e.g. 10M.

Kali arsenicum 6c   Pruritis aggravated by warm conditions. Fissuring in the bends of the joints. Dose: night and morning for one week.

Sulphur iodatum 6c   When there is danger of a secondary infection occurring. Dose: night and morning for ten days.

Thuja 200c   Long-standing cases. There may be enlargement of associated glands. Dose: once daily for two weeks.

Hydrocotyle 6c   This remedy often gives success when the better known remedies fail to act. Dose: night and morning for ten days.

11.   Acne.   Infection of hair follicles by a special bacillus or by any pyogenic bacterium e.g. staphylococcus. A non-specific form is common in the horse and lesions can occur in pressure areas e.g. under the saddle.

SYMPTOMS
Lesions commence as nodules quickly becoming pustular and spreading to other neighbouring follicles.

TREATMENT
Hepar sulphuris 200c   It is probable that this remedy, given where the symptoms are uncomplicated, may have to be repeated in increasingly higher potencies. First dosage: night and morning for one week.

Sulphur iodatum 6c   Associated eczema with redenning of skin. Dose: night and morning for one week.

Arsenicum alb. 1M   When skin is dry and itchy. Animal restless and thirsty. Dose: once daily for ten days.

Silicea 200c   Sweats easily, with lesions which coalesce quickly and penetrate the subcutaneous tissues. Dose: once daily for two weeks.

Kali bromatum 6c   When lesions affect shoulder and head. Skin is insensitive to pain. Dose: night and morning for one week.

Ledum 6c   Acne associated with facial eczema. Itching made worse by warmth. Dose: night and morning for one week.

Hydrocotyle 6c   Pustules worse on the chest, associated with skin desquamation and severe itching. Dose: night and morning for one week.

Antimonium crudum 6c   Warty excresences and dry skin. Hard scabs appear over the pustules. Dose: night and morning for five days.

12.   Sporotrichosis – Mycotic Dermatitis.

This is a contagious disease of horses caused by a specific fungus. It leads to the development of nodules on the skin and ulceration of the lower limbs. The disease may be spread either by direct contact, or through contaminated bedding or harness.

SYMPTOMS
Groups of small nodules develop on the skin of the legs particularly about the fetlock. The nodules develop scabs which discharge pus, but they are usually painless. The condition has a tendency to spread and form new nodules and there may, or may not, be an associated lymphangitis.

TREATMENT

Sepia 30c Useful in fungal conditions. Dose: once daily for two weeks.

Bacillinum 200c In mycotic conditions, this is a very good remedy. Dose: once weekly for three doses.

Arsenicum alb. 1M An excellent skin remedy and can often be combined with other treatment. Dose: once daily for ten days.

Calcarea iodata 200c When the condition is combined with swellings of the associated glands. Dose: once daily for five days.

Silicea 200c When the nodules discharge pus and the ulcers are slow to heal. Dose: once daily for one week.

13. Ringworm. Ringworm lesions in the horse may be superficial or deep, the former being the more common, producing desquamation and alopecia with development of thick crusts.

SYMPTOMS

Irritation and itching may first occur, the lesions developing initially on the rump and trunk and spreading to other parts. When deeper structures are involved, small suppurative foci develop in the hair follicles, producing a small scab over the follicles.

TREATMENT

Hydrocotyle 6c When there are scaly lesions on the trunk. There is exfoliation of scales of the skin. Dose: night and morning for one week.

Bacillinum 200c Rough, dry skin. Give as a constitutional remedy. Dose: once per week for three doses.

Sepia 1M Associated with unpleasant musty odour. Dose: once a week for four doses.

Pix liquida 6c Tendency to alopecia. Eruptions scaly and itchy. Dose: night and morning for one week.

14. Sebaceous Cysts. Occasionally these occur in the horse, being sited mainly on the sheath and the false nostril and the lips. The cysts contain fatty material along with dead cells and are due to the retention of sebaceous material in the glands. They are usually soft and fluctuating in the early stages, but may become firm and doughy later. Inflammatory symptoms appear if the cyst is subject to constant irritation.

TREATMENT

Baryta carb. 30c   Cysts prominent on the head and face. Dose: twice daily for five days.

Benzoic acid 6c   Cysts on face, accompanied by cystitis with dark offensive urine. Dose: three times daily for five days.

Conium 200c   Long standing cases when cysts are usually firm and hard. Dose: once daily for seven days.

Apis 30c   Early stages when there is an abundance of fluid present and inflammatory symptoms appear. Dose: every three hours for four doses.

XIV Affections of the Female Reproductive System

1. Infertility. Hormone dysfunction can occur frequently in the form of cystic ovaries, and ovaritis without cyst formation. Leucorrhoea, endometritis and vaginitis also occur.

Ovaritis. Inflammation of the ovary may lead to irregularities in ovarian function and can result in extension of inflammation to oviducts and the formation of adhesions in the ovarian bursa.

SYMPTOMS
The mare exhibits signs of pain in the pelvic area, kicking at one or other of the flanks. Temperament may change, e.g. a normally docile animal may become difficult. Rectal examination reveals an increase in the size of the ovary concerned.

TREATMENT
Aconitum napellus 6c   Early acute stage. Febrile signs – rapid, firm pulse and increased respiration. Dose: hourly for four doses.

Apis 6c   Inflammation with swelling due to hyperaemia leading to oedema. Dose: three times daily for two days.

Bryonia 6c   Right ovary affected, shown by animal kicking at right pelvic flank. Animal prefers to be still and quiet. Dose: three times daily for two days.

Lilium tigrinum 200c   Accompanying signs of uterine inflammation such as discharges. Hind legs weak, frequent straining movements. Dose: three times daily for three days.

Cimicifuga 30c   Left ovary affected. Pains extend across lumbar region and downwards towards the udder. Heart action weak and irregular. Dose: night and morning for four days.

Hamamelis 6c   General venous congestion with this complaint.

Blood vessels of throat usually enlarged. Pain extends over whole abdomen and there may be a metrorrhagia. Dose: three times daily for three days.

Iodum 6c   Thin animals showing excessive appetite and dryness of skin. Mammary glands appear shrunken. Dose: three times daily for one week.

Cantharis 30c   Furious excitement and severe strangury. Urine contains blood and is passed drop by drop. Vesication of skin may occur. Dose: two hourly for four doses.

Palladium 30c   Right ovary affected, with leucorrhoea and flatulence. Dose: night and morning for one week.

2. Cystic Ovaries.   This condition is associated with an over-development of the Graffian follicle and its persistence in the ovaries. It may be associated with an absence of heat or, at the other extreme, a state of nymphomania may occur. Between these extremes are signs of irregular heat. The condition sometimes resolves itself, but when extreme, the enlarged follicle becomes filled with fluid and is referred to as cystic.

SYMPTOMS
In mares which do not show heat periods, there are usually one or two large cysts present. These are detected by rectal palpation. Mares showing cystic ovaries are usually uncertain in temperament. When the condition occurs in animals which show continuous or irregular lengthy heat periods, multiple small cysts develop and a state of nymphomania supervenes.

TREATMENT
Apis 6c   As one of the main remedies for dropsical conditions, this should be tried as an initial treatment. Dose: three times daily for four days.

Aurum mur. nat. 6c   When a chronic metritis is suspected, and whitish discharge shows. Ovaries may be indurated. Dose: three times daily for four days.

Colocynth 6c   Nymphomania, with multiple small cysts. Symptoms of great abdominal pain. Dose: night and morning for one week.

Oophorinum 6c   Accompanying skin disorder, e.g. a non-pruritic eczema. Dose: three times daily for one week.

Platina metallicum 30c   Nymphomania, with constipation and abdominal pain extending to pelvis. Dose: night and morning for one week.

Aurum iodatum 6c   Accompanying degenerative lesions in other areas, e.g. chronic inflammatory conditions of serous membranes. Dose: three times daily for one week.

3. Leucorrhoea. This condition implies a whitish mucoid, catarrhal or purulent discharge from the vulva. It may be associated with increased activity of the uterine glands and usually has its origin in ovarian dysfunction when there is failure to ovulate despite good follicular activity.

SYMPTOMS

There is passive non-inflammatory bland discharge from the vulva, usually whitish and mucoid. Secondary infection of the uterine mucous membrane leads to a purulent discharge. If the discharge becomes acrid, the skin around the vulva becomes excoriated.

TREATMENT

Pulsatilla 30c   Discharge acrid, thick and creamy. Urinary symptoms such as pain during and after micturition. Dose: night and morning for five days.

Alumen 30c   Chronic state. Discharge has yellow colour and there may be necrosis of areas of the vagina. Dose: night and morning for one week.

Hydrastis 30c   Discharge bland and catarrhal. Mucous membranes elsewhere may also show this type of discharge. Dose: three times daily for five days.

Kali muriaticum 6c   Discharge bland and milky-white. There may be accompanying glandular swellings and a thick white-coated tongue. Dose: night and morning for one week.

Kreosotum 30c   Discharge greenish-yellow and acrid, has a pungent odour. There may be swellings and ecchymotic haemorrhages on the skin. Dose: night and morning for one week.

Nitric acid 6c   Vaginal mucous membrane ulcerated and there is brown, watery discharge. Small ulcers may also appear in the mouth. Dose: once daily for one week.

Psorinum 1M   Harsh dirty coat showing rough eczematous patches. Skin has heavy, musty odour. Discharge contains lumps of mucous material and there are signs of weakness, especially along the back muscles. Dose: once daily for five days.

Thuja 200c   Wart formation on various parts of the body, especially round the vulva. Discharge thick and greenish. Dose: once a week for one month.

4.   Endometritis.   This is commonly associated with a difficult parturition or with retained foetal membranes especially after abortion. These conditions cause a delay in involution of the uterus which leads to the metritis.

SYMPTOMS
There is a vulval discharge which at first is mucoid, but soon becomes purulent, due to secondary bacterial invasion. The inflammation extends to the anterior area of the vagina and produces a thickened corrugated condition of the uterine cervix and vagina. Febrile symptoms in acute cases following protracted labour or retention of foetal membranes following abortion. These signs include rapid, wiry pulse, shallow respiration and sweating. Signs of pain include kicking at the flank and looking round to the pelvic area. Straining is a common symptom.

TREATMENT
Aconitum napellus 6c   Give early in the acute febrile stage. Animal anxious and restless. Dose: hourly for four doses.

Belladonna 1M   Acute cases, when there is full pulse, dilation of pupils and a hot, smooth skin. Dose: every two hours for four doses.

Echinacea 6x   Puerperal fever, or septicaemia sets in after abortion or retention of unhealthy foetal membranes. Dose: two hourly for four doses.

Sabina 6c   Discharge of bright blood, partly clotted. Especially useful if condition results from abortion. Urine blood-stained. Dose: three times daily for four days.

Secale 30c   Puerperal metritis after abortion, where discharge of blood is dark and fluid. Dose: three times daily for four days.

Arsenicum alb. 200c   Chronic endometritis in restless animals, showing thirst for small quantities. Worse after midnight. Dose: one dose daily for ten days.

Mel cum sale 6c   Chronic endometritis when cervix is particularly affected and at commencement of inflammatory process. Dose: three times daily for three days.

Sulphur 200c   This can usefully be given in chronic cases, in combination with other indicated remedies. Dose: one dose weekly for three days.

Note:—   As this condition is frequently associated with streptococcal infection, it will be found profitable to combine treatment with the use of Streptoccocus nosode, giving one dose per day for three consecutive days at the beginning of treatment.

5.   Vaginitis.   Inflammation of the vagina can arise as a sequel to or complication of coitus and parturition. It is also seen in mares when a heat period coincides with a feverish illness such as influenza.

SYMPTOMS

The vaginal mucous membrane becomes red and thickened and a mucous discharge appears which becomes purulent, due to secondary infection. Straining is a common sequel.

TREATMENT

Aconitum napellus 6c   Febrile signs accompanying the acute phase. Dose: every two hours for three doses.

Hydrastis 30c   Discharge is catarrhal and bland. There may be catarrh of other mucous membranes. Dose: three times daily for two days.

Cantharis 200c   Severe urinary symptoms: urine is passed drop by drop and contains blood. Mare strains violently and kicks at lower abdomen. Dose: every two hours for four days.

Mercurius sol. 30c   Secondary purulent discharge, greenish and streaked with blood. Slimy blood-stained stools and salivation. Dose: three times daily for three days.

Pulsatilla 30c   Discharge bland and creamy. Signs of colic. Dose: three times daily for three days.

Nitric acid 200c   Ulceration on posterior vagina. Discharge thin, watery and brown. Possibly mouth ulcers and diarrhoea. Dose: night and morning for four days.

Arsenicum alb. 200c   Discharge acrid and burning, excoriating skin round vulva. Mare restless, thirsty, worse after midnight. Dose: three times daily for three days.

6. Abortion. This can arise from various causes, some of which are specific and are dealt with under specific diseases. Non-specific causes include injuries and over-exertion and may also follow an attack of severe colic.

SYMPTOMS
The signs are those of approaching parturition, viz. loosening of the sacral and pelvic ligaments, discharge of blood-stained fluid, kicking at abdomen and general restlessness. The pulse is quickened and becomes firm and wiry.

TREATMENT
Aconitum napellus 6c   Give immediately on first signs of impending abortion. Dose: every hour for four doses.
Arnica 30c   Abortion results from injury. Dose: every three hours for three doses.
Opium 200c   Abortion resulting from severe fright. Dose: twice in one day only.
Secale 200c   Will help control post-abortion haemorrhage when accompanied by much straining. Blood dark and clotted. Dose: every three hours for four doses.
China off. 30c   Much loss of blood, with great weakness. Dose: every two hours for four doses.
Sabina 6c   Hamorrhage, with bright red blood, partly clotted. Dose: every three hours for four doses.
Pyrogenium 1M   Septic abortion associated with retention of foetal membranes, producing a low grade fever characterised by discrepancy of pulse and temperature, e.g. a weak thready pulse with high temperature, or a full pulse with low temperature. Dose: every three hours for four doses.
Note:—   Treatment should always be directed towards the associated effects such as retained placenta, endometritis, uterine discharge, etc.

7. Retained Placenta.   This is not a common occurrence in the mare, but may occur occasionally after a normal parturition. It is more commonly seen after abortion and can be accompanied by severe symptoms such as laminitis and septicaemia. Normally the foetal membranes are expelled shortly after parturition but if not expelled after two hours one or other of the following remedies should be given:—

Sabina 6c   Dose: every hour for four doses.
Pulsatilla 30c   Dose: every three hours for three doses.
Secale 30c   Dose: every two hours for three doses.
Pyrogenium 1M   Dose: every three hours for three doses.

8.   Inflammation of Udder.   This may arise in a nursing dam, due to exposure to cold and sometimes as a result of an inability on the part of the foal to suck enough milk.

SYMPTOMS
There may be an initial febrile involvement, such as rapid pulse and increased respiration. The mouth may be hot and constipation is usually present. Local symptoms include heat and tenderness of the gland which is swollen and firm in acute cases. Softening of the swelling is accompanied by the formation of cheese-like curds which may contain blood.

TREATMENT
Expression of the contents of the udder should be accompanied by the use of one of the following: —
Aconitum napellus 6c   Early in febrile symptoms. Dose: every hour for four doses.
Phytolacca 6c   Associated lymph glands are involved. Udder swollen and tender. Dose: three times daily for two days.
Belladonna 1M   Acute case, excitability, dilated pupils, full bounding pulse. Udder hot and swollen. Dose: every two hours for four doses.
Bryonia 6c   Gland hard, but less hot than when Belladonna is indicated. Dose: three times daily for three days.
Hepar sulphuris 200c   Suppuration, udder extremely tender, mare resents touch. This remedy in low potency, e.g. 6x will hasten expression of purulent material, but in higher potency, will hasten resolution. In either case, one dose three times daily for two days, of the appropriate potency, should suffice.
Mercurius sol. 30c   Secretion greenish, blood-stained. Udder tissue firm after evacuation of contents. There may be an accompanying blood-stained diarrhoea. Dose: three times daily for three days.
Silicea 200c   When superficial ulcers appear and are slow to heal, showing thin, creamy pus. Dose: once daily for five days,

S.S.C. 30c   This is a combination of *Sulphur, Silicea and Carbo veg.* and may be used to ease expression of clotted milk. Dose: three times daily for three days, followed by one dose daily for three days.

XV Affections of the Musculo Skeletal System

1. Myopathy. This term implies degeneration of muscle tissue, non-inflammatory in origin. A common form in saddle horses is the condition known as polymyositis.

SYMPTOMS
The affection shows clinically as muscle weakness. It can develop suddenly during exercise and can lead to necrosis of muscle tissue of the hind quarters. The skeletal muscles become rubbery and swollen and the animal moves with a short, painful gait, or may be disinclined to move at all.

Myopathy has been reported in the thoroughbred foal up to about four months of age, appearing in spring or early summer. A per-acute form exists in which dejection, stiffness and disinclination to move are the chief symptoms. Less acute cases may move more readily but are stiff and lethargic. The subcutaneous tissues over the gluteal muscles become swollen and firm and this occurs also at the base of the mane. Excessive salivation has been noted, also superficial ulceration of the tongue.

TREATMENT
Sarcolactic acid 30c   Muscles of the neck and back affected. Muscular prostration and possibly dyspnoea. Dose: night and morning for four days.
Picric acid 6c   Muscular weakness and involvement appear to deteriorate in an ascending manner. Symptoms worse after motion. Dose: night and morning for one week.
Thuja 200c   Sweating accompanied by twitching of muscles. Dose once daily for one week.
Cuprum metallicum 1M   Cramping accompanies a general hardening of muscles. Dose: once daily for one week.

2. **Muscular Spasm.**   Spasm of muscle may take one of two forms: (a) tonic or continuous spasm, and (b) clonic or intermittent. The former can occur in such diseases as tetanus, but can also arise after prolonged exertion and may appear up to twelve hours after discontinuing exercise. Clonic spasms are more usually associated with poisoning or certain nervous diseases.

SYMPTOMS

Arnica 30c   After prolonged or violent exercise. Dose: every three hours for two doses.

Cuprum metallicum 1M   Clonic spasms accompanied by cramping of muscles. Dose: hourly for four doses.

Agaricus muscarius 6c   Twitching, with cramp-like condition of lower limbs. Dose: every two hours for four doses.

Strychninum 200c   Pronounced clonic spasm of any muscle group. Dose: every two hours for four doses.

Cicuta virosa 6c   Extensive tonic spasms. Muscles of nape of neck and head chiefly involved. Dose: every three hours for four doses.

Strophanthus 6c   Clonic spasms, especially muscles of the upper part of the body. Dose: every two hours for four doses.

Cimicifuga 30c   Heaviness of lower limbs accompanied by twitching. The animal is usually restless and shows signs of pain. Dose: every three hourly for four doses.

3. **Rupture of Muscles.**   Muscle rupture may result from excessive contraction and relaxation and may involve associated tendons. Violent injury or strain may also lead to rupture.

SYMPTOMS

Inflammation and swelling are early signs, the latter often due to extravasated blood. Lameness will be evident if limb muscles are involved.

TREATMENT

Arnica 30c   All cases. Dose: every two hours for two doses.

Ruta graveolens 30c   If there is an associated rupture of tendon at its insertion. Dose: three times daily for three days.

4. **Myositis.**   Inflammation of muscle tissue may have its origin in an open wound or in infection, or it may be the result of severe straining.

SYMPTOMS

Local heat in the muscle is an early sign, followed by stiffness or lameness if leg muscles are involved. Febrile signs will accompany infectious conditions.

TREATMENT

Arnica 30c   Should always be given in the early inflammatory stage. Dose: every two hours for two doses.

Apis 6c   Oedema accompanies inflammation. Dose: every three hours for four doses.

Hepar sulphuris 30c   Infection from an open scratch or wound. Dose: three times daily for three days.

5.   Muscular Atrophy.   Wasting of muscle tissue may follow myositis or be dependent on an impaired nerve supply.

SYMPTOMS

These are obvious, comprising reduction in muscle size and loss of muscular function.

TREATMENT

Arnica 30c   All cases, in as much as injury of one kind or another has been the original cause. Dose: every two hours for two doses.

Gelsemium 200c   Local paralysis of nerve supply, provided there has been no permanent damage. This remedy helps loss of nerve function. Dose: three times daily for three days.

Curare 30c   Muscular paralysis associated with trembling of limbs and various groups of muscles. Dose: three times daily for four days.

Lathyrus sativa 200c   Atrophy of gluteal muscles and those of stifle and hock. Dose: three times daily for five days.

Plumbum 1M   Generalised paralytic involvement leads to affection of various groups of muscles. Feet often become swollen. Extensor muscles are more involved when this remedy is indicated. Dose: once daily for seven days.

Thallium 30c   Paralysis of lower limbs leading to atrophy. Evidence of recurring pains. Dose: twice daily for five days.

Abrotanum 6c   Marked wasting of the lower limbs, accompanied by stiffness of joints. Dose: three times daily for four days.

Acetic acid 6c   Wasting of muscles accompanied by oedema of feet and legs. Dose: twice daily for seven days.

6.   Osteodystrophy.   This term implies failure of normal bone development, or abnormal growth of already developed bone.

SYMPTOMS

The main symptom is distortion and enlargement of bones and susceptibility to fracture. Gait is interfered with. Rickets of young animals and Osteomalacia of adults are manifestations, caused by deficiencies of calcium, phosphorus and vitamin D. A spondylitis occurs in the horse and can affect racing performance. It is thought by some authorities to start as a disc degeneration. Weakening of bones leads to fractures and deformities depending on the age of the animal. Bony enlargements occur especially at the ends of large bones.

TREATMENT

Calcarea phosphorica 200c   Signs of pain accompanying enlargements at ends of long bones. This remedy has given excellent results in young animals. Dose: once daily for two weeks.

Phospheric acid 6c   Debility in young, growing animals. Periostium frequently affected. Dose: night and morning for one week.

Iodum 30c   Painful enlargements of joints, with dry, withered-looking skin. Dose: once daily for one week.

7.   Osteoarthritis.   Degenerative lesions of joint cavities, non-inflammatory in origin are grouped under this heading. These lesions can accompany bone diseases such as osteodystrophy.

SYMPTOMS

In affections of limbs, lameness occurs and in severe cases there is distension of joint capsule together with crepitus. The articular surfaces of the cervical vertebrae are sometimes affected in the horse. This may cause pain and difficulty of movement. More frequently compression of spinal nerves is the cause rather than the affection of the bone itself. Involvement of the stifle joint may lead to fracture of the head of the tibia causing complete recumbency. When the hip joint is affected reduction in the head of the femur takes place.

TREATMENT

Osteoarthritis nosode 30c   This remedy may help alleviate some of the painful symptoms. Dose: once a week for four doses.

Rhus toxicodendron 1M   Amelioration of symptoms of pain when the animal moves. Dose: once daily for one week.

8.   Arthritis.   This condition differs from osteoarthritis in being inflammatory in origin, commonly bacterial. In new-born foals a common cause is Salmonella abortus-equi.

SYMPTOMS

Pain, stiffness, heat and swelling occur, due to inflammation of the synovial membrane. The hock, stifle and carpus are the joints chiefly affected, while in foals involvement of several joints is common, leading to severe lameness and recumbency.

TREATMENT

Apis 6c   In the early stage, when the joint is swollen and there is an increase in synovial fluid. Dose: every two hours for four doses.

Rhus toxicodendron 30c   Lameness improved by exercise. There may be an associated stiffness of muscles and tendons. Dose: night and morning for four days.

Belladonna 200c   Joints are very hot and swollen without excess of joint fluid. Various joints may be simultaneously affected. The animal is usually excitable. Dose: every two hours for four doses.

Bryonia 30c   Pressure over joints relieves. The animal is worse on movement. Dose: night and morning for four days.

Note:—   Brucellosis is a disease which has now become recognised as a cause of bacterial arthritis in the horse, e.g. in the atlanto-occipital bursa, the navicular bursa and the vertebral joints of the withers. Before commencing any of the above remedies, it would be helpful to administer one dose of the *Brucella abortus nosode 30.*

XVI Affections of Bursae

1. **Acute Bursitis.** Bursa is the term generally employed to include all synovial sacs and refers to the true bursa situated between tendon and bone, or between two tendons and also includes joint capsule and synovial sheath. Bursitis may be dry, serous or purulent and arises as a result of open wound infection or contusion.

SYMPTOMS
The dry form quickly leads to the serous or purulent forms. There is a swelling at the particular site which contains either clear, serous fluid or purulent material.

TREATMENT
Bryonia 30c In the initial inflammatory stage, there is relief from pressure and symptoms are worse on movement. Dose: every three hours for four doses.
Apis 6c Excess of fluid formed by inflammation. Dose: every two hours for four doses.
Hepar sulphuris 200c Purulent bursitis. Extreme tenderness and sensitivity to touch. Dose: every three hours for four doses.

2. **Chronic Bursitis.** This may take the form of a cystic swelling or of a fibrous enlargement. It may follow the acute form or arise independently. The cystic form contains a clear fluid while the fibrous form is firm and contains only a small amount of fluid.

SYMPTOMS
Distension and enlargement are the only prominent signs and there is evidence of lameness or pain.

TREATMENT

Calcarea fluorica 30c   Swelling. This remedy, given over a long period is beneficial. Dose: twice daily for seven days, followed by one dose weekly for three week.

Apis 6c   Cystic form, with excess fluid. Dose: twice daily for seven days.

XVII Bacterial Diseases

A. Streptococcal

1. Strangles. This disease is usually accute and is characterised by upper respiratory tract inflammation together with
abscess formation in the sub-maxillary glands. Young animals are
principally affected. There is a high incidence when groups of
horses are exposed to inclement conditions.

SYMPTOMS
The disease commences with fever and nasal discharge, at first
mucoid, but soon becoming purulent. Cessation of feeding
occurs. Throat involvement is usual, in the form of an acute
lymphadenitis. A persistent moist cough is present in most cases.
The temperature, high in the initial stage, usually falls in two to
three days, but may recur once abscesses develop in the throat
glands. These become hot, swollen and tender to touch.
Accompanying this abscess formation is an increase in purulent
nasal discharge. The abscesses may rupture, discharging a thick,
creamy pus. Extension to neighbouring lymph glands is the
rule in severe cases, while accumulation of pus in the guttural
pouches can result from neglected cases. Metastatic spread of
infection results in complications such as pneumonia and arthritis.

TREATMENT
Aconitum napellus 6c   Always the first choice remedy in early
    febrile stage. If given early enough, this remedy alone may
    bring about resolution of the disease. Dose: hourly for four
    doses.
Belladonna 1M   Full bounding pulse, dilated pupils, nervous
    excitability. Dose: every two hours for four doses.
Phytolacca 30c   Neighbouring lymph glands or salivary glands
    in the throat become firm, tender and swollen. Dose: three

times daily for four days.

Pulsatilla 6c   Yellow mucous discharge from nose. Pharyngeal area tender. Dose: night and morning for three days.

Mercurius sol. 200c   Salivation and possibly slimy diarrhoea. Nasal discharge oily and greenish, possibly blood-stained. Dose: night and morning for three days.

Hepar sulphuris 200c   Low potencies will help abscesses to mature. In higher potency, condition will be aborted without rupture of the abscesses. Dose: low potency, e.g. 6x, three times daily for one day. Higher potency: night and morning for two days.

2.   Neo-natal Streptococcal Infection.   S. pyogenes is frequently involved in infection of the umbilicus, resulting in bacterial spread to other organs, especially the joints. The source of the infection is contamination by uterine discharges from an infected mare, the infection presumably taking place through the umbilicus. Septicaemia sets in from the patent umbilicus producing suppurative lesions throughout the body. Although arthritis is the most usual complication, ophthalmia can also develop in foals which are affected when they become two to three weeks old.

SYMPTOMS

Initially there is swelling and pain of the umbilicus and there is usually an oedematous plaque surrounding the navel. Patent urachus is common and there may be a purulent discharge from the umbilicus. Febrile symptoms are slight. The joints commonly affected are the hock and stifle and occasionally the carpus. Lameness may be severe and recumbency is common.

TREATMENT

Streptococcus Nosode 30c   This nosode should always be employed. Sometimes it will be curative by itself. Dose: once daily for three days, followed by one dose every second day for three doses.

Apis 6c   Synovitis severe. Joints puffy, tender to touch. Dose: every two hours for four doses.

Rhus toxicodendron 1M   Arthritis, when animal improves on movement. Dose: three times daily for three days.

Benzoic acid 6c   Indicated when the carpus is involved. Accompanying tenderness and swelling of the Achilles tendon. Urine dark brown, offensive. Dose: three times daily for two days.

Bryonia 6c   Joints swollen, hot and tender. Pain better from pressure, symptoms worse on movement. Dose: three times daily for three days.

Lycopodium 200c   Shoulder and elbow joints affected. Accompanying sweating of the limb and possibly hepatic symptoms. Dose: night and morning for three days.

Natrum phosphoricum 30c   When the carpus is especially involved. Affected joints show crepitation. Dose: night and morning for one week.

Note:—   Prevention of this condition is possible, by administering the nosode to the in-foal mare, giving one dose per month for the last four months of pregnancy, followed by two doses in the last week. This will help to mitigate symptoms in the young animal and possibly prevent infection entirely, as it is thought by some authorities that intra-uterine infection can occur. An additional preventive measure is to give the foal one dose of nosode immediately at birth and repeat every day for four days.

3.   Genital Tract Infection of Mares.   Streptoccal infections of the genital tract can occur in mares and show usually as metritis, which can lead to abortion and sterility. Coitus is thought to be the cause of its spread.

SYMPTOMS
Metritis in the acute stage is evidenced by fever and signs of toxaemia. The pulse rate is increased, respiration is more rapid and sweating is common. Systemic involvement may lead to laminitis. The inflammation in the uterus may extend to the vagina producing a corrugated thickening and a vulval discharge at first mucoid, later purulent. If abortion occurs retention of foetal membranes follows. Chronic metritis may lead to sterility and is associated with changes in the endometrium accompanied by chronic discharges.

TREATMENT
Streptococcus nosode 30c   Always commence treatment with this remedy. Dose: three times daily for two days.

Aconitum napellus 6c   Early stages of acute infection. Dose: every hour for four doses.

Exhinacea 6x   Puerperal involvement follows the metritis. Dose: every two hours for four doses.

Pyrogenium 1M   Metritis resulting from abortion. Retention of foetal membranes. Rapid, thready pulse in contrast to a low temperature, or weak faint pulse and high temperature. Dose: every three hours for four doses.

Sabina 6c   Haemorrhages of bright blood from the uterus. Retained foetal membranes. Dose: every hour for five doses.

Belladonna 1M   Mare excitable, with dilated pupils, full bounding pulse, sweating and hot skin. Dose: every two hours for four doses.

Sepia 200c   Chronic metritis. Intermittent uterine discharge. Dose: once weekly for four doses.

Hepar sulphuris 6c   Purulent involvement in chronic cases. Dose: three times daily for five days.

4.   Ulcerative Lymphangitis of Foals.   This is a streptococcal disease affecting foals only and is distinct from the commoner lymphangitis associated with corynebacteria occurring in older animals.

SYMPTOMS

Swelling of lymphatic vessels occurs and neighbouring lymph glands show firmness, if the condition is very acute. Normally, however, there is only slight involvement of these glands. The lymphatics become corded due to the development of abscesses. When these mature and burst, ulceration of the lymphatic vessels occur discharging pus of a creamy, thick nature. The surrounding tissue becomes swollen due to cellulitis.

TREATMENT

Streptococcus nosode 30c   Give once daily for three days.

Silicea 200c   Ulceration having occurred, this remedy will rapidly heal the abscess and resolve necrotic tissue. Dose: night and morning for three days.

Hepar sulphuris 6x-200c   In low potency, abscess material will be expelled, while the higher will abort the process. Dose: three times daily for two days of potency 6x, or one dose night and morning for three days of potency 200c.

B. Corynebacterial Infections

1. Contagious Acne – Contagious Pustular Dermatitis. This disease is characterised by the development of pustules in pressure areas, caused by C. pseudotuberculosis. Spread from animal to animal is by infected grooming utensils or harness.

SYMPTOMS
The hair follicle is first affected, leading to local suppuration and eventually pustular formation. There is an initial papular lesion which is sometimes painful, but not itchy, and this develops into a pustule which eventually ruptures, liberating a greenish pus.

TREATMENT
Arsenicum alb. 1M Thirst, restlessness, worse after midnight. Lesions sometimes attended by local oedema. Dose: once daily for one week.
Antimonium crudum 6c Accompanying gastric symptoms. Itching made worse by warmth. Dose: three times daily for three days.
Hepar sulphuris 200c Tendency to suppuration. Dose: night and morning for five days.
Sulphur 6c This is a good general remedy to be used as a constitutional aid to elimination of toxins from the blood and may profitably be combined with other remedies. Dose: night and morning for three days.
Sulphur iodatum 6c Inter-current throat affections. Skin surrounding lesions is red and itchy. Dose: night and morning for ten days.

2. Corynebacterial Pneumonia of Foals. This disease of young foals produces pneumonia and respiratory lesions generally and is caused by C equi. It is a frequent cause of death in breeding stables and most commonly affects animals one to two months old, but may cause illness in foals up to six months old.

SYMPTOMS
There is an initial fever which is caused by a bacteraemia leading to development of suppurative lesions in various organs but particularly the lungs. The younger the animal, the more severe the clinical symptoms. Pneumonia develops quickly in these

cases, accompanied by lesions in the joints, causing an acute arthritis. In older animals, a moist cough leads to a slowly developing pneumonia and emaciation. The animal may continue to suck, but gradually loses condition. Profuse diarrhoea often accompanies the respiratory disease. Upper respiratory involvement is uncommon.

TREATMENT

Aconitum napellus 6c   In the initial febrile stage. Dose: every hour for four doses.

Arsenicum alb. 6c   The older foal showing emaciation, restlessness, frequent thirst, dry skin and diarrhoea. Dose: three times daily for one week.

Antimonium tartaricum 30c   Moist cough, with rattling mucus and dyspnoea. Dose: three times daily for four days.

Lycopodium 200c   Laboured breathing involving the alae nasi and accompanied possibly by liver symptoms. Dose: night and morning for one week.

Phosphorus 200c   Rapid onset, blood-stained cough which contains fibrinous shreds. Dose: three times daily for two days.

Arsenicum iodatum 30c   When the more severe conditions have been resolved, this remedy will aid recovery. Dose: once daily for one week.

Tuberculinum aviare 200c   Young animals showing acute broncho-pneumonia with weakness and debility. Dose: once daily for four days.

3.   Ulcerative Lymphangitis.   This is a contagious disease caused by C. pseudo-tuberculosis, infection due to scratches on the lower limbs. It can spread quickly when horses are grouped together in large numbers.

SYMPTOMS

Beginning with skin infection, spread takes place to the lymphatic vessels, producing abscesses along their course. Swelling of the pastern usually follows initial infection, frequently producing lameness. Subcutaneous nodules appear over the fetlock area and eventually discharge a creamy pus, sometimes green tinged. The ulcer which develops becomes indolent and necrotic. The lymphatic glands associated with the area become infected and fresh abscesses and ulcers develop, producing hardening and thickening. The disease can persist for many months in untreated cases.

TREATMENT

Calcarea fluorica 30c   Lymph glands and vessels are hard, before suppuration begins. Dose: three times daily for three days.

Phytolacca 200c   Lymph glands swollen and hot. Dose: night and morning for five days.

Silicea 200c   Chronic cases, when ulcers tend to spread and become fistulous. Indolent ulcers and necrotic patches will heal quickly under this remedy. Dose: once daily for five days.

Hepar sulphuris 6x-200c   Lower potencies of this remedy hasten maturation of abscesses. Higher potencies resorb the condition. Dose: three times daily for one day of potency 6x, and one dose night and morning for two days of potency 200c.

C. Clostridial Disease

1.   Tetanus.   This disease is caused by the bacillus Cl. tetani, which produces a toxin which has a predilection for nervous tissue. The toxin is formed in deep punctured wounds which have become infected by the tetanus bacillus. The organism can produce the toxin only in the absence of free oxygen, hence the liability of the disease to show after the occurrence of a deep wound in the susceptible animal. An idiopathic form of the disease also occurs in which there is no observable wound, infection probably taking place from an internal wound.

SYMPTOMS

After an incubation period of one to three weeks, there appears a general stiffness of all muscles accompanied by muscle tremors. Clamping of jaws supervene and prolapse of the third eyelid occurs. The tail is held straight out behind the body. The expression is invariably tense and alert with retraction of the lips and erect positioning of the ears. There is exaggerated response to stimuli. Constipation and retention of urine are present and there is inability to feed or open the mouth. In prolonged cases there is arching of the back and tetanic convulsions eventually appear along with opisthotonus and extreme extension of the limbs. Sweating may be profuse along with marked pyrexia. Death occurs by paralysis of respiration.

TREATMENT

Animal should be kept in darkened loose-box, in absolute quiet.

Aconitum napellus 6c   If seen early enough after the initial injury and also during the febrile stage, should there be one. Dose: every hour for four doses.

Belladonna 1M   Great excitement, dilated pupils, full bounding pulse, skin hot and smooth. Dose: every two hours for four doses.

Nux vomica 1M   Stiffness of limbs and constipation severe. Dose: every four hours for four doses.

Ledum 6c   When origin of disease is a deep, punctured wound and is *not* idiopathic. Give immediately wound is sustained. Dose: every two hours for three doses.

Hypericum 1M   Damage to nerve endings. The remedy will prevent infection ascending the nerve paths. It should be combined with Ledum in alternate doses. Dose: every two hours for three doses.

Strychninum 200c   When tetanus spasms and muscle rigidity first appear. This remedy alone has been known to effect a cure if the disease process has not advanced too far. Dose: three times daily for one week.

Arnica 30c   Since the source of the disease is not only injury, but is accompanied by shock, give early in the course of the disease – two doses four hours apart.

Tetanus nosode 30c   Give early in course of disease. It will aid action of other remedies. One dose daily for five days.

2. **Botulism.**   This condition is essentially a motor paralysis caused by the absorption from the stomach or intestine of the toxin of Cl. botulinum. It is usually sub-acute in the horse and produces a picture of progressive muscular paralysis.

SYMPTOMS

The muscles affected are usually those of the limbs, jaw and throat. Weakness and paralysis commence in the hind quarters and ascends to the forelegs and head region. Stumbling and knuckling occur and there is inability to raise the head. The animal later becomes recumbent with its chest on the ground

and head turned towards the flank. Paralysis of the tongue causes
it to protrude from the mouth. Involvement of the chest muscles
produces a laboured abdominal breathing.

TREATMENT
This should always begin with the administration of the Cl.
botulinum nosode and should be given three times daily for
three days.
Conium 30c   Conditions showing ascending paralysis. It may
   be necessary to give ascending potencies at short intervals.
   Dose: three times daily for three days.
Gelsemium 200c   Weakness and paralysis of the head region.
   Dose: three times daily for two days.
Plumbum metallicum 200c   Paralysis may be accompanied by
   a cold feeling of lower limbs and associated with bouts of
   colic. Dose: night and morning for five days.

D.   Salmonellosis

1.   Paratyphoid Disease.   Disease caused by Salmonella usually
takes the form of an acute septicaemia or an acute or chronic
enteritis. The chief organism concerned is S. typhimurium and
foals are principally affected. Adult horses which are overfed
prior to transport are also susceptible.

SYMPTOMS
Septicaemic symptoms are seen in young foals, producing fever
and depression. This form may produce early fatalities. An
enteric form is associated with dysentery or diarrhoea according
to the severity of the infection. Shreds of intestinal mucous
membrane may be evident in the faeces. Thirst is prominent and
acute abdominal pain is nearly always present. Polyarthritis is
a common sequel to the disease in foals.

TREATMENT
Salmonella Typhimurium Nosode 30c   This should be given
   three times daily for two days at the beginning of treatment.
Mercurius sol. 200c   Stools slimy and dysenteric, often worse
   during the night. Dose: three times daily for two days.
Baptisia 30c   Thin, dark stools often blood-stained with tenderness over the abdomen. Dose: three times daily for three days.

108   THE TREATMENT OF HORSES BY HOMOEOPATHY

Camphor 30c   Threatened collapse. The body surface is cold. Dark watery stools. Dose: every two hours for four doses.

Veratrum album 6c   Watery diarrhoea accompanied by pain. Stools forcibly evacuated, followed by prostration. Dose: three times daily for three days.

Arnica 30c   Congestive venous states accompany blood-stained putrid stools. Dose: three times daily for two days.

Arsenicum alb. 1M   Restlessness, worse at night, thirst for small quantities. Dose: three times daily for three days.

2.   Salmonella Abortion in Mares.   This infection, caused by S. abortus equi is confined to horses and donkeys. Natural infection can occur from ingestion of contaminated feed, usually from uterine discharges from other mares, while transmission by coitus is thought probably also. Infection can persist in uterus and cause subsequent abortion.

SYMPTOMS

Infection by ingestion leads first to a bacteraemia, the bacteria subsequently becoming lodged in the placenta, resulting in abortion. Less virulent infection can result in viable first term foals but these may be infected, disease being spread via the umbilicus. Abortion usually occurs at about seven or eight months and is accompanied by difficult expulsion of the foetus. Retention of foetal membranes and metritis are common sequelae.

TREATMENT

Caulophyllum 200c   The entire process of pregnancy can be usefully controlled by this remedy. Dose: once a month until the final month, when the dose should be one dose at two-weekly intervals.

Sabina 6c   If abortion has occurred, this remedy will help to reduce discharges and also to expel the placenta. Dose: every hour for four doses.

Secale 30c   Post-abortion discharges, contaminated by dark-coloured blood will be helped by this remedy. Dose: every four hours, for one day.

3.   Testicular Lesions.   S. abortus equi has been implicated in testicular lesions in the stallion, leading to oedema of the prepuce, followed occasionally by orchitis and atrophy of testicular tissue. Arthritis may also occur.

TREATMENT

Salmonella abortus equi nosode 30c   This should be used as a preliminary to the use of other remedies. Dose: daily for five days.

Belladonna 1M   Acute orchitis, with excitability and dilated pupils, full bounding pulse, testicles swollen and hot. Dose: once daily for five days.

Rhododendron 6c   Testicular lesions indurated, left testicle being more involved. Dose: three times daily for three days.

Spongia 6c   Testicular swelling extends to the epididymis. Pain and tenderness in testicles. Dose: three times daily for three days.

Aurum metallicum 30c   Testicular swelling is long-lasting leading eventually to induration. Dose: night and morning for one week.

Pulsatilla 30c   Testicular swelling extends along the abdomen, with urethral discharge. Dose: night and morning for five days.

Apis 6c   Oedema of the prepuce prominent. This remedy will also reduce testicular swelling when due to oedema. Dose: three times daily for two days.

XVIII Miscellaneous
Bacterial Infections

Among the conditions which are important to consider are Brucellosis, E. coli infection, Shigella Disease of Foals and Leptospirosis.

1.   Brucellosis.   In the horse the organism Brucella abortus has been associated with bursitis of various joints, poll evil, and fistulous withers being considered prominent examples. The sacro-iliac joint is one that is frequently affected and lameness in this joint should be considered as possibly due to brucellosis. Some authorities have recently attributed the inflammation of the navicular bursa to this organism. Arthritis of the lower joints is also thought to be due to brucellosis, leading to intermittent lameness and transient fever. This disease can also cause hygromatus swellings on the skin which may yield a honey-coloured viscid fluid arising from numerous small vesicles.

TREATMENT

Brucellosis abortus and Brucellosis Melitensis nosode 30c   The combined use of these nosodes is always indicated at the beginning of the course of treatment. Dose: night and morning for three days.

Hepar sulphuris 30c   As brucellosis is a pyogenic infection, the use of this remedy invariably produces good results, especially when the condition is accompanied by extreme sensitivity to cold and wind. Pain and tenderness exist over affected areas such as fistulous withers. Dose: every three hours for four doses. It may be necessary to continue treatment at regular intervals with ascending potencies.

Silicea 200c   The more chronic and neglected case, when abscess formation has taken place, the underlying tissue having become necrotic leading to fistulae. Dose: once daily for seven days.

Apis 6c   Acute synovitis, joint showing tenderness, swelling and heat. Dose: every two hours for four doses.

Rhus toxicodendron 1M   Joint ligaments involved, with improvement on exercise. Dose: night and morning for one week.

Bryonia 6c   Acute swelling and firmness of joints. Worse on movement. Dose: three times daily for three days.

2.   E. Coli Infection. Colibacillosis.   The septicaemic form of this infection is the more usual, although arthritis can be a common sequel in foals which recover.

SYMPTOMS

There is usually a cold skin and sub-normal temperature, slowness of heart and signs of impending coma in the very acute type. Less acute cases show depression, weakness and increased heart rate. The initial high temperature falls and diarrhoea sets in. This takes various forms and ranges from watery to pasty consistency and may be tinged with blood. The stool has a characteristic rancid odour and soils the buttocks. Abdominal signs include colic and kicking at belly and there may be tympany and tenesmus.

TREATMENT

E. coli nosode 30c   The use of this nosode has given good results, a peculiarity being that it does not have to be prepared from the particular strain of organism concerned in the illness. Experience has shown that nosode made from many different strains is effective. Dose: three times daily for two days.

Arsenicum alb. 6c   Diarrhoea is watery and tinged with blood. Animal restless, thirsty, worse after midnight. Dose: three times daily for three days.

Ipecacuanha 30c   Less acute cases, when faeces less watery, slimy, green. Dose: three times daily for two days.

Colchicum 6c   Signs of tympany appear, with signs of colic. Dose: every two hours for four doses.

Colocynth 6c   Should be considered when severe abdominal pain is evident. Animal rolls and looks round at flanks. Dose:

every hour for four doses.

China off. 6c   Profuse watery stools. Great weakness. Dose: every two hours for four doses.

Mercurius corrosivus 200c   Disease takes the form of severe enteritis, with passage of slimy blood-stained stools, accompanied by salivation. Stools more frequent during night. Dose: three times daily for two days.

3.   Shigella Disease of Foals.   This is an acute septicaemic disease of foals, particularly the new-born. It is limited to horses. Foals may contract infection through the umbilicus, or become infected *in utero.*

SYMPTOMS

Suppurative lesions develop internally in animals which survive an acute attack. An early symptom is a febrile reaction and increased respiration. Diarrhoea and dysentery may occur. Foals frequently show comatose or sleepy symptoms. Arthritis develops in animals which survive acute attacks.

TREATMENT

Aconitum napellus 6c   Give in early febrile stage. Dose: every hour for four doses.

Arsenicum alb. 1M   Enteric symptoms. Diarrhoea usually acrid and has carrion-like odour. Straining, with restlessness and thirst. Dose: three times daily for two days.

Rhus toxicodendron 1M   Arthritis cases which show improvement on movement. Joints hot and stiff. Dose: night and morning for three days.

Note:—   A nosode could be prepared from the causative organism *Shigella equirulis* which could be cultured from the stool of infected foals. This nosode would be a useful complement to other indicated remedies.

4.   Leptospirosis.   This infection, due to leptospira species is usually mild in the horse, although occasionally blindness has resulted, possibly as a result of an associated ophthalmia.

SYMPTOMS

There is an initial fever and a degree of haemoglobinuria. Jaundice is a fairly common sequel and abortion may follow.

TREATMENT

Aconitum napellus 6c   Give in the early febrile stage, one dose hourly for three doses.

Chelidonium 30c   Jaundice, with tenderness or lameness over right shoulder region. Dose: night and morning for three days.

Berberis vulgaris 30c   Haemoglobinuria   present.   Tenderness over lumbar region. Dose: three times daily for four days.

XIX Virus Diseases

1.   Infectious Equine Anaemia.   This is a contagious disease of horses which produces a chronic illness, caused by a specific virus which attacks all age groups. The disease is usually confined to summer and autumn and shows an incubation period of two to four weeks.

SYMPTOMS
Early signs are depression, incoordination and rapid wasting. Febrile symptoms are intermittent and follow an undulating pattern. Petechial haemorrhages appear on the conjunctiva while jaundice and oedema become evident. The heart's action is increased and the sound is intermittent. Epistaxis may occur and an increase in the size of the spleen may be felt on palpation. Relapses are common, leading to further emaciation and weakness. There may be a watery diarrhoea, but it is an inconstant sign. Abortion may occur.

TREATMENT
There is no specific treatment, but the following remedies will produce alleviation of symptoms:–

Aconitum napellus 6c   In the early febrile involvement. Dose: every hour for four doses.

Phosphorus 200c   Petechial haemorrhages occur on mucous membranes. Dose: three times daily for three days.

Chelidonium 20c   Jaundice. Possible stiffness over right shoulder area. Dose: night and morning for four days.

Apis 6c   In oedematous states, this remedy will help control the amount of fluid in the tissues. It will have to be combined with other indicated remedies. Dose: three times daily for two days.

China off. 6c   Great loss of strength in anaemic states. Dose: three times daily for three days.

Note:— If possible, a nosode should be made from infected blood drawn from the patient about the fifteenth day after infection, when the febrile reaction is usually at its height. Such a nosode could be used both prophylactically and theraputically.

2. African Horse Sickness. This disease has recently spread to Europe. It is caused by various species of virus and follows an acute, mild or chronic course. The incubation period is from five to seven days.

SYMPTOMS
The acute type takes a pulmonary form producing an initial fever, dyspnoea and coughing. Nasal discharge of yellow frothy material occurs, followed by sweating and incoordination of gait. The mild or sub-acute type has a longer incubation period of up to three weeks and symptoms develop more slowly. Oedema of the head region is the main outward sign, showing particularly on the eyelids and lips and may spread to the pectoral region. Petechial haemorrhages are seen under the tongue, and the mouth shows a bluish colour. Hydropericardium is common in the more chronic type and endocarditis may occur. Pulmonary oedema, if it occurs, is dependent on the weak heart action. Sometimes the cardiac and pulmonary forms co-exist, one type developing into the other.

TREATMENT
Aconitum napellus 6c   In the early febrile stage. Dose: every hour for four doses.
Antimonium tartaricum 30c   Pulmonary signs, showing dyspnoea and coughing. Dose: three times daily for three days.
Apis 6c   Oedematous state. This remedy will control the amounts of fluid present in the pulmonary and cardiac forms. Dose: three times daily for two days.
Kali bichromicum 200c   Yellowish discharge from nose. Dose: three times daily for three days.
Phosphorus 200c   Petechial haemorrhages on mucous membranes. Dose: three times daily for two days.
Conium 200c   Incoordination of gait and weakness of hindquarters. Dose: three times daily for three days.
Note:—   A nosode can be made from infected blood, the virus

being present in the blood-stream from the first day of clinical illness. It could be used both prophylactically and theraputically.

3.   **Vesicular Stomatitis.**   This is an infectious disease caused by a virus producing crops of vesicles on the mouth and feet.

SYMPTOMS
A primary viraemia develops and localisation takes place in the mucous membranes of the mouth and the skin around the coronet. The lesions in the horse are more usually found in the mouth, on the dorsum of the tongue, or on the lips. The external genital organs can also show involvement. When the vesicles rupture, a ropy saliva is produced.

TREATMENT
Aconitum napellus 6c   When the primary viraemia sets in, this remedy will be useful in controlling the febrile reaction. Dose: every hour for three doses.
Antimonium crudum 6c   Tongue heavily coated and eczema appears round the mouth. Dose: three times daily for three days.
Borax 6c   When vesicles appear both in the mouth and above the coronet. The animal is disinclined to move. Dose: three times daily for four days.
Natrum muriaticum 200c   Dry mouth and vesicles extend to the lips. Dose: night and morning for three days.
Argentum nitricum 30c   Papillae of tongue unduly prominent. There may be bleeding from the gums. Dose: night and morning for four days.
Nitric acid 200c   Associated ulcers on soft palate. Tenderness of feet. Vesicles appear mainly on the sides of the tongue. Dose: night and morning for four days.
Kali muriaticum 30c   Aphthous whitish ulcers develop. Slimy coating on tongue. Dose: three times daily for three days.

4.   **Equine Viral Rhinopneumonitis.**   This disease of the upper respiratory tract may also cause abortion and is usually mild in character, although abortion may be of frequent occurrence if the disease appears among brood mares. Transmission is by droplet infection or ingestion of contaminated material. Carrier

animals are common and are a frequent cause of continued spread of the disease. The incubation period is two to ten days.

SYMPTOMS

The pregnant uterus becomes infected after an initial viraemia. Infection of the respiratory tract causes rhinitis and interstitial pneumonia, followed by pyraemia, conjunctivitis and coughing. Submaxillary lymphadenitis may occur. Some months after respiratory involvement, abortions may occur, shedding of the placenta taking place with the expulsion of the foetus. There is pronounced leucopenia.

TREATMENT

Aconitum napellus 6c   If seen early enough in the initial viraemic state, give one dose hourly for four doses.

Kali hydriodicum 200c   Conjunctivitis, cough and pulmonary oedema. Dose: three times daily for three days.

Antimonium tartaricum 30c   Interstitial pneumonia with moist cough and rattling of mucus. Dose: night and morning for three days.

Arsenicum alb. 200c   Animal restless, thirsty and has foul-smelling diarrhoea. This remedy will help associated rhinitis and pneumonia. Dose: every two hours for four doses.

Phytolacca 200c   Cases showing lymphadenitis. Dose: three times daily for four days.

Caulophyllum 30c   The use of this remedy will be found helpful in regulating pregnancy and allaying the tendency to abortion. Dose: once a month of pregnancy, with two doses during the last month.

Viburnum opulus 6c   Another useful remedy in controlling abortion. Dose: once a week for the first three months.

Note:—   A nosode could be made from any infective material and employed as an oral vaccine and also theraputically.

5.   Infectious Equine Pneumonia.   This virus disease produces a severe lobar pneumonia accompanied by septicaemic complications. It may arise when large numbers of horses are brought together from different regions.

SYMPTOMS

Primary virus involvement is fairly mild, but secondary bacterial invasion produces the severe symptoms. Lobar pneumonia follows a primary viraemia. The incubation period may be as long as thirty days, associated with fever and increased heart rate. Respiratory signs come later accompanied by sanguineous nasal discharge. Consolidation of lung tissue soon follows along, with exudation. Moist rales are heard on auscultation and harsh friction sounds are heard over the pleura.

TREATMENT

Aconitum napellus 6c   Early febrile stage. Dose: every hour for four doses.

Phosphorus 200c   Hepatisation. Severe dyspnoea with rust-coloured nasal discharge. Dose: three times daily for three days.

Antimonium tartaricum 30c   Moist cough and mucous rales. Dose: night and morning for four days.

Bryonia 6c   Pleuritic involvement. Pressure on chest relieves. worse on movement. Dose: three times daily for two days.

Lycopodium 200c   Symptoms worse late afternoon. There may be signs of liver involvement, jaundice. Dose: night and morning for five days.

Ferrum phosphoricum 6c   Blood coughed up. Symptoms appear better at night. Dose: three times daily for three days.

Iodum 6c   This remedy may be useful when condition is accompanied by a dry withered look of the skin. Animal worse in warmth and seeks cool air. Dose: three times daily for three days.

Sanguinaria 6c   Nervous animals showing dilation of blood vessels, easy sweating and blood-stained rust-coloured mucus when coughing. Dose: three times daily for three days.

6.   Equine Viral Arteritis.   This disease is characterised by an acute upper respiratory tract infection and abortion. The small arteries show specific lesions. The chief economic significance is loss of foals due to abortion and mares of all age groups are susceptible. Infection is presumed to be air-borne or by ingestion of contaminated material.

SYMPTOMS

After an incubation period of up to six days fever develops and a muco-purulent nasal discharge takes place. Conjunctivitis and lachrymation are common sequelae. Cough and pulmonary congestion occur leading to severe dyspnoea. Vascular damage occurs to small arteries and a haemorrhagic arteritis develops causing diarrhoea or dysentery. Pulmonary and limb oedema occur and occasionally jaundice. Abortions in this disease occur much earlier than in equine viral rhinopneumonia and differ also in that there are no lesions in the foetus. The vascular lesions produce a haemorrhagic picture in many of the internal organs, petechiae being present on most of the serous surfaces.

TREATMENT

Aconitum napellus 6c   Give early in the febrile stage, one dose hourly for four doses.

Arsenicum alb. 1M   Rhinitis and diarrhoea. Animal is restless, thirsty. Dose: every two hours for four doses.

Kali hyrdiodicum 200c   Conjunctivitis and lachrymation. Pulmonary oedema. This is one of the remedies most likely to alleviate symptoms. Dose: three times daily for four days.

Antimonium tartaricum 30c   Moist cough accompanies pulmonary congestion. Mucous rales prominent. Dose: three times daily for three days.

Phosphorus 200c   Petechial harmorrhage, liver involvement and jaundice. Dose: three times daily for three days.

Millefolium 6c   General haemorrhagic diathesis with tendency to continued febrile involvement. Dose: three times daily for three days.

Apis 6c   This remedy will help to control oedema. Dose: three times daily for two days.

Crotalus horridus 30c   This remedy also will help control a haemorrhagic tendency especially purpura-like ecchymosis and will have value in controlling uterine involvement. Dose: three times daily for three days.

7. **Viral Encephalomyelitis.** This is an infectious disease characterised by derangement of consciousness leading to paralysis after an initial motor irritation. Infection in horses is accidental from birds and spread is by vector, possibly mosquitoes and ticks.

SYMPTOMS

Viraemia is common to begin with and may be transitory or persistent according to the strain of virus. The incubation period is one to three weeks and initial symptoms are fever and depression. Hypersensitivity is the earliest nervous sign and disturbances of vision soon follow. Involuntary muscle twitching occurs. Somnolent states are common as the disease progresses, Paralysis is the rule and when the mouth is affected, the tongue protrudes. Incoordination of gait is common and the disease may progress to total paralysis.

TREATMENT

Aconitum napellus 6c Give early in viraemic stage, one dose every hour for four doses.

Hyoscyamus 30c Will help control hypersensitivity and early nervous signs. Dose: three times daily for three days.

Agaricus muscarius 6c Vertigo and depression. Dose: three times daily for three days.

Strychninum 200c Muscular twitchings and chorea prominent. Dose: three times daily for three days.

Opium 200c Somnolent state associated with paralysis of bowel movement. Dose: twice in twenty-four hours.

Plumbum meallicum 30c General paralytic state, worse at night. Extreme hyperaesthesia, associated with bouts of pain. Dose: night and morning for four days.

Gelsemium 200c Paralytic involvement of head and tongue are the most prominent symptoms. Dose: three times daily for two days, followed by one dose weekly of potency 1M for three weeks.

Conium 30c Ascending paralysis, starting in the hind legs. Dose: three times daily for three days. It has sometimes been found necessary to use ascending potencies after an interval.

8. Borna Disease.

This is an infectious encephalomyelitis caused by a virus which is fairly resistant to environmental factors. The incubation period is up to one month.

SYMPTOMS

Febrile signs are slight and hyperaesthesia and muscle tremors occur. Swallowing becomes difficult owing to paralysis of the throat region. Lassitude and general paralysis takes place.

TREATMENT

Hyoscyamus 30c   Hyperaesthesia, with head shaking. Naturally excitable animals will benefit from this remedy. Dose: three times daily for three days.

Strychninum 200c   Muscular twitching and chorea, with tendency to muscular rigidity. Dose: three times daily for three days.

Gelsemium 200c   Motor paralysis prominent in throat region, making swallowing difficult. Dose: night and morning for three days.

Conium 200c   Paralysis affecting hindquarters and limbs, showing a tendency to ascend. Dose: night and morning for four or five days.

Agaricus muscarius 6c   Lassitude, hyperaesthesia and vertigo. Dose: three times daily for three days.

9. Horse Pox.   This condition is usually benign and is characterised by typical pox lesions on the limbs and on the lips. Badly affected animals may lose condition severely.

SYMPTOMS

The lesion commences as a small papule and progresses to vesicle, pustule and scab formation. When the leg is affected, the lesions are usually seen on the back of the pastern. Those on the mouth form on the buccal mucosa. Lameness may supervene and stomatitis may develop.

TREATMENT

Thuja 200c   This will help resolve the lesions and promote rapid healing of scabs without scarring the skin. Dose: once daily for one week.

Antimonium crudum 6c   Scab formation is accompanied by a honey-coloured secretion. Itching may occur towards night. Dose: night and morning for one week.

Borax 6c   Lesions develop into ulcers on the palate, producing stomatitis. Dose: night and morning for five days.

Nitric acid 200c   Ulceration of the soft palate, with diarrhoea and ulceration of the external genitals. Dose: night and morning for five days.

10.   Papillomatosis.   Warts of this nature are caused by a virus. In the horse they are usually confined to the muzzle, nose and lips and are invariably sessile.

TREATMENT

Thuja 200c   This is the main remedy for papillomatous warts, especially those which bleed easily. Dose: once daily for ten days.

Causticum 30c   This remedy may be indicated for hard warts associated with weakness and tremors of the foreleg muscles. The warts are usually worse on the nose. Dose: night and morning for one week.

Calcarea carbonica 200c   Warts small, hard and do not bleed easily. Dose: once daily for one week.

XX   Protozoal Diseases

1. **Babesiasis.**   This disease is characterised by fever and intravascular haemorrhage or haemolysis producing an anaemic state,
along with haemoglobinuria. The causative organism is transmitted by ticks.

SYMPTOMS
An initial pyrexia is followed by anorexia and weakness. The
conjunctivae are at first bright red, but soon become pale due to
anaemia. Jaundice may supervene in the later stages. Mares if
pregnant may abort. Haemoglobinuria is rare in the horse, but
oedema of various parts is common, e.g. in the supraorbital
fossa. Colic and petechial haemorrhages on the conjunctiva have
been observed.

TREATMENT
China off. 6c   This is a good supportive remedy in anaemic
    states, helping to maintain strength and control pyrexia. Dose:
    every two hours for four doses.
Ferrum arsenicum 6c   Enlarged spleen, accompanied by dry
    skin. Dose: night and morning for one week.
Phosphorus 200c   Petechial haemorrhages. Dose: night and
    morning for four days.
Silicea 1M   This remedy has some reputation in restoring red
    cells and stimulating haemopoiesis. Dose: once weekly for
    four weeks.

2. **Dourine.**   This contagious disease is caused by *Trypanosoma
equiperdium,* a flagellate protozoon. It is transmitted by coitus
and affects principally the external genital organs. It produces
lesions also on the skin and in some cases paralysis.

SYMPTOMS

Local oedematous swellings occur after initial infection and systemic involvement follows. The incubation period may be up to one month and sometimes longer. Swelling of the penis and scrotum are the first signs in the stallion and the oedema may extend forward as far as the pectoral region. Urethral discharge occurs and there is involvement of the regional lymph nodes.

Vulval oedema occurs in the mare accompanied by vaginal ulceration and discharge. As in the stallion the oedema spreads downwards and forward. Nervous symptoms appear in both sexes leading to incoordination of movement, and in the later stages, paralysis, preceded by atrophy of the hindquarters. In severe cases there may be sexual excitement and more severe oedema. Skin lesions in the form of plaques appear over the neck and various parts of the body.

TREATMENT

Apis 6c   Oedema of genitalia. Oedematous plaques on skin. Dose: three times daily for five days.

Urtica urens 6c   Itch accompanies formation of oedematous areas. Dose: three times daily for five days.

Rhus toxicodendron 1M   Scrotal skin becomes erythematous and itchy with initial swelling. Dose: three hourly for four doses.

Conium 200c   Paralysis. This remedy helps to prevent hind-quarter atrophy. Dose: night and morning for one week.

3.   **Coccidiosis.**   This contagious disease takes the form of an enteritis caused by a protozoon parasite, *Eimeria leukarti.* Characteristic of the condition is dysentery, followed by emaciation and anaemia. The disease may affect a group of young animals, if they are kept in close confinement, e.g. foals running together in a paddock. Animals become infected by ingestion of contaminated feed or water.

SYMPTOMS

After a variable incubation period of fourteen to twenty-one days, a mild febrile reaction occurs. Diarrhoea, usually severe, is the first noticeable sign, the faeces containing mucus and whole blood, sometimes dark, but more often bright red. This is accompanied by severe straining which can persist long after faeces are passed. If much blood is lost in the stool, signs of anaemia occur, e.g. paleness of mucous membranes and conjunctivae, together with weak, rapid pulse and general weakness. Appetite is lost and dehydration sets in. Mild cases may show only diarrhoea and stunted growth, without loss of blood.

TREATMENT

Aconitum napellus 6c   Signs of fever in early stages of the disease. Dose: every hour for three doses.

Arsenicum alb. 1M   First stage of diarrhoea, especially if faeces are evil-smelling and worse after midnight. Dose: every two hours for four doses.

Ipecacuanha 30c   Protozool infection of the intestine. Faeces contain abundant mucus, shreds of mucous lining and whole blood, usually bright red. Dose: three times daily for three days.

Millefolium 6c   Accompanying haemorrhages from urinary tract and from the nose. Dose: three times daily for three days.

China off. 30c   Great loss of strength after loss of blood. Dose: three times daily for two days.

Mercurius corrosivus 200c   Stools bloody, excessively slimy, passed more often during the night. Dose: three times daily for three days. This remedy is particularly useful for straining unaccompanied by stool.

XXI Miscellaneous Diseases

1. **Haemolytic Anaemia of New Born Foals.** The predisposing factors of this disease occur during pregnancy, but the foetus is not affected. Symptoms show only after birth when the young animal has ingested colostrum. The foal inherits red cell antigens from the sire and these pass the placental barrier into the dam's circulation. If these antigens are not normally present in the dam, antibodies are produced in the dam's circulation against the foal's red cells. These antibodies are produced late in pregnancy, but do not pass the placental barrier, so the foetus remains unaffected. The antibodies against the foal's red cells are present also in the dam's colostrum and are soon absorbed into the foal's circulation after it has sucked for the first time. These produce intravascular haemolysis because of the interaction of antibody and red cells resulting in anaemia and jaundice.

Vaccination against rhinopneumonitis has been suggested as a possible cause, especially if this is done twice during pregnancy in the last three months, using a vaccine which has been prepared from foetal tissue.

SYMPTOMS
Clinical signs appear only if the colostrum has been ingested and are evident after two to four days in the average case. There may be per-acute, acute or sub-acute involvement. Early signs include lassitude and disinclination to suck, the foal usually lying on its chest, The heart rate is increased and the cardiac sounds are intensified, having a metallic tone. A jugular pulse is evident. Once anaemia develops, respiration becomes laboured and yawning is frequent. Haemoglobinuria is present in per-acute cases, jaundice being absent. Sub-acute cases show a reversal of these two findings.

TREATMENT

Replacement of affected blood in the foal by transfusion is normal practice and is usually effective. The following remedies will aid recovery:—

China off. 30c   This remedy will quickly help the foal to regain strength and regulate heart and respiration. Dose: every two hours for four doses.

Phosphorus 200c   This remedy will help to promote a healthy peripheral circulation and restore liver function. Dose: three times daily for two days.

Note:—   If there is cause to believe that this disease may arise because of a history of pneumonia vaccination, the above remedies should be given to the foal immediately at birth, prior to having the affected blood replaced by transfusion. Replacement of orthodox or allopathic vaccination by a nosode or homoeopathic oral vaccine will reduce the likelihood of the disease occurring.

2.   **Purpura haemorrhagica.**   This is a non-contagious disease characterised by oedematous and haemorrhagic swellings in the subcutaneous tissues. Mucosal and visceral harmorrhage also occur. It frequently follows an attack of an infectious disease such as strangles, infectious arteritis or pneumonitis. The incidence is highest where there are large numbers of horses at risk in an outbreak of strangles.

SYMPTOMS

Subcutaneous swellings characterise the initial stages of the disease; these are oedematous and are seen particularly around the muzzle and lips. They are painless and may appear suddenly or over the course of a few days. Oedema of the limbs is confined to areas above the knee or hock. Oozing of serum may take place from the swellings. Petechial haemorrhages occur on the conjunctiva and submucous harmorrhages in the mouth and nasal passages. Colic may occur due to visceral oedema and haemorrhage. The heart rate is increased but the temperature usually remains normal.

TREATMENT

Apis 6c   This remedy should be employed as soon as oedematous swellings first appear. Dose: every two hours for four doses.

Phosphorus 200c   This is indicated for petechial haemorrhages. It will also help visceral haemorrhages especially if hepatic in origin. Dose: three times daily for three days.

Kali bichromicum 30c   This will prevent further development of oedematous swellings. It is also useful in controlling the oozing of serum from swellings. Dose: three times daily for three days.

Crotalus horridus 200c   This is a valuable remedy for general haemorrhagic diathesis, with oozing of dark blood from petechial haemorrhages. It is particularly useful if jaundice is present. Dose: four times daily for two days

Lachesis 30c   This remedy may be indicated when generalised petechial haemorrhages are accompanied by throat swelling and epistaxis. Dose: three times daily for three days.

Hamamelis 6c   This is an important remedy. There is a generalised venous congestion with enlarged throat veins. Purpura and petechiae are accompanied by pain. Dose: three times daily for three days.

Sulphuric acid 30c   This remedy is especially useful if the condition has arisen as a result of strangles. Petechiae are associated with a skin irritation. Dose: three times daily for three days.

If there is a history of previous infectious disease, the appropriate nosode should be administered at the commencement of treatment. It may be combined with indicated remedies. Dose: once daily for three days.

3. **Allergic Dermatitis.**   This extremely itchy condition is due to a hypersensitivity to insect bites. The majority of cases occur during the summer months, especially if the weather is humid. The condition is confined to horses and all ages are affected. Stabled animals clear themselves of the condition. Affected areas are the base of the tail, the rump, along the back to the withers and forward to the ears.

SYMPTOMS

Pruritis is intense and is worse at night. Constant scratching causes shedding of the hair and secondary infection may occur in the hair follicles. In mild cases, the skin may appear scaly with loss of hair.

TREATMENT

Arsenicum alb. 30c This is one of the main remedies. It may have to be given in progressively high potencies. Dose: once daily for ten days.

Sulphur iodatum 6c This is useful in long standing cases, showing a tendency to secondary infection. Dose: three times daily for one week.

Hepar sulphuris 200c This is indicated when the hair follicles have become infected and localised suppuration has occurred. It is especially useful if the lesions are tender to the touch. Dose: night and morning for one week.

Mezereum 30c This remedy will be found useful in neglected cases where scab formation has developed around the lesion. Dose: three times daily for two days, followed by one dose daily for five days.

4. Fistulous Withers. This is the term applied to a sinus or fistula which develops along any part of the withers. As in poll-evil abscess formation and necrosis affect the ligamentum nuchae in this region, but involvement of spinous processes and cartilages is also of common occurrence. When bone is involved the lesion is carious.

SYMPTOMS

An extremely tender inflammatory swelling of the withers occurs. Various openings discharge purulent material and the disease tends to move downwards and forwards, affecting deeper tissues. Secondary septicaemic involvement is common, with febrile symptoms.

TREATMENT

Aconitum napellus 6c If seen early enough, this should be given to prevent febrile complications. Dose: every hour for three doses.

Apis 6c This remedy is indicated to control synovitis which may occur in the small joints involved. Dose: every two hours for four doses.

Hepar sulphuris 200c This is a most useful remedy, the guiding principle being extreme sensitivity to pain, which almost always is present in the acute stage. This remedy will also help once suppuration has occurred, promoting resolution and relieving pain. Dose: three hourly for four doses.

Silicea 200c   This remedy is indicated in more neglected cases, once fistulae have appeared. Its use will prevent necrosis and promote healthy granulation of ulcers. Dose: once daily for seven days.

Brucella abortus nosode 30c   As brucellosis is frequently implicated in this disease, the nosode should be given for three consecutive days at the commencement of treatment. Dose: once daily.

Externally, a lotion of *Calendula* and *Hypericum* will promote quick healing and aid the action of indicated remedies.

5.   Poll Evil.   This condition is a bursitis, affecting the atlanto-occipital joint, leading to necrosis of the ligamentum nuchae and resulting in a sinus or purulent fistula of the poll region.

SYMPTOMS

Heat, tenderness and swelling of the area first occur, the joint becoming extremely sensitive to touch. Secondary infection leads to suppuration which tends to invade the surrounding tissues and may infect adjacent bone. Fistulous involvement occurs, caused by necrosis of tissue in the ligamentum nuchae.

TREATMENT

Brucella abortus nosode 30c   This nosode should be given at the commencement of treatment. Dose: once daily for three days.

Aconitum napellus 6c   This remedy should be given in the early febrile stage. Dose: every hour for four doses.

Apis 6c   If synovitis of the joint is suspected, in the acute stage, this remedy will relieve pain and reduce the joint fluid. Dose: every two hours for four doses.

Hepar sulphuris 30c   This remedy will be of considerable benefit if given either in the early inflammatory stage, showing extreme sensitivity to pain, or when suppuration has set in. Dose: every two hours for four doses.

Silicea 200c   This is a valuable remedy in the more chronic case, once fistulous involvement has occurred with the development of purulent channels. Dose: once daily for seven days.

Externally, a compress of *Hypericum* and *Calendula* lotion will hasten healing.

6. Leuco-encephalomalacia. This condition is sometimes seen as a result of horses feeding on mouldy corn, which arises as a result of wet grain being stored allowing moulds to develop.

SYMPTOMS
Early signs of disturbance include weakness accompanied by tremors of various groups of muscles. The animal may walk in circles and staggering and incoordination may appear. The reflexes become sluggish, while abdominal disturbance is manifested by jaundice in a proportion of cases. Febrile signs are absent.

TREATMENT
Agarius muscarius 6c   This remedy will help those cases showing depression of consciousness and incoordination of movement. Dose: every two hours for four doses.
Curare 30c   This remedy is indicated in the early stages showing muscle weakness and tremors. Dose: hourly for four doses.
Plumbum metallicum 30c   When the main symptom is walking in circles, with a tendency to paralysis, this remedy should help. Dose: three times daily for one week.
Phosphorus 200c   The administration of this remedy will help liver function and control petechial haemorrhages which may occur in some parts of the central nervous system. Dose: every three hours for four doses.
Chelidonium 1M   This is a useful remedy when there is jaundice, accompanied by muscle stiffness over the right shoulder area. Dose: three times daily for three days.

7. Snake Bite. The adder-type of bite causes a local swelling and severe pain. Dyspnoea can arise from bites near the throat. Other types of bite may produce vesicular involvement leading to haemorrhages and secondary infections.

SYMPTOMS
The area surrounding the bite becomes swollen and discoloured, sometimes assuming a bluish or purplish appearance.

TREATMENT
Apis 6c   This remedy is indicated for adder bites when accompanied by local oedema. Dose: three times daily for two days.

Naja 6c   This remedy will be of use when underlying tissue oedema is accompanied by purplish discolouration of the skin above. There is usually much salivation. Dose: every two hours for four doses.

Crotalus horridus 200c   Indications for this remedy include haemorrhage and localised secondary infection. The blood is dark and fluid. Dose: every two hours for four doses.

Echinacea 6x   Indicated when there is secondary infection from venous wounds. This takes the form of blood poisoning with involvement of lymphatics. Dose: every hour for five doses.

Tarentula cubensis 6c   This remedy will be useful when there is a puffy swelling round the bite, with early suppuration. The underlying skin is purplish. Dose: every two hours for four doses.

Lachesis 1M   When the skin surrounding the wound appears bluish, with systemic symptoms involving the region of the throat, this remedy will be found to be useful. Dose: hourly for four doses.

Anthracinum 200c   This nosode is indicated when the subcutaneous tissues become indurated and necrotic. The blood is dark, with the associated lymph glands becoming swollen and tender. Dose: every two hours for four doses, followed by one dose daily for three days.

8.   Calcium Deficiency.   This may occur among horses during training, if kept indoors for much of their time, and is usually associated with vitamin D deficiency.

SYMPTOMS

Signs are commoner in the young animal and show usually in retardation of growth and poor or abnormal development of teeth. In older animals anorexia, stiffness and a tendency to recumbency occur, together with a predisposition to fracture of the long bones.

TREATMENT

Calcarea phosphorica 30c   The most useful remedy for restoring a healthy, calcium metabolism. Dose: night and morning for two weeks.

9.   Osteodystrophia Fibrosa.   In this condition fibrous tissue is deposited in place of calcium, which becomes deficient due to excessive phosphate feeding. It can be induced by Ca: P. ratio of one to three or more. Diets which contribute to this condition include cereal hay, together with heavy grain or bran feeding. The imbalance of calcium and phosphorus produces a demineralisation of bone, leading to a susceptibility to fractures and separation of the attachment of muscles and tendons.

SYMPTOMS
Lameness appearing in different legs is the first obvious sign and there may be an arching of the back. Joint lesions sometimes occur, producing a crackling sound when the animal moves. Different parts of the skeleton produce their own picture of involvement, e.g. the facial bones may become swollen and the ribs flattened. Joint swellings and bending of long bones are seen in advanced cases.

TREATMENT
Calcarea phosphorica 30c   This is the remedy which should be tried first, helping as it does to restore the calcium and phosphorus ratio. Dose: night and morning for two weeks.
Calcarea fluorica 30c   Where joint exostoses and any dental involvement occur, this is the remedy of choice. Dose: night and morning for seven days. This is a form of treatment which may have to be repeated at monthly intervals.
Phosphoric acid 6c   The young, rapidly growing animal responds well to this remedy. Dose: once daily for ten days.

10.   Copper Deficiency.   Primary copper deficiency is rare in adult horses, but foals may show abnormalities of the limbs, if reared in copper deficient areas. Such animals, if untreated, usually remain unthrifty and slow growing.

SYMPTOMS
Enlargement of joints and stiffness are early signs. The flexor tendons are subject to contraction, shown by the animal putting the toe to the ground when walking. Severe cases may show knuckling.

TREATMENT
Cuprum metallicum 200c   This remedy should be administered once a day for one week, followed by a dose twice weekly for four weeks.

11.   Iodine Deficiency.   Deficiency of this element may be primary, produced by an insufficient intake, or it may be secondary when it is then associated with too much calcium in the feed.

SYMPTOMS

Iodine deficiency assumes its greatest importance as a main contributory cause of still births, or weakly viable foals. This weakness may be severe enough to prevent the foal standing unaided. The fetlock and pastern areas of the fore limbs sometimes show excessive flexion, coupled with a corresponding extension of the same areas in the hind leg. Thoroughbreds and hunters in affected areas may show thyroid enlargement in the adult animal.

TREATMENT

Iodum 6c   This should be given twice daily for one week, but it may be necessary to continue treatment for longer periods, depending on response.

Kali hydriodicum 12x   The iodide of potassium is a more suitable preparation for weakly foals, influencing, as it does, the extremities. Dose: twice daily for seven days.

12.   Horsetail Poisoning.   This may occur from time to time, as a result of young or immature plants being incorporated into a hay crop. Animals rarely show symptoms when grazing.

SYMPTOMS

Incoordination of movement, along with swaying from side to side are early signs. The hind legs may be splayed out and crossing of the fore legs is not uncommon. Muscle tremors arise, followed by arching of the back, leading to recumbency. Coma may eventually set in, preceded by opisthotonus and possibly brain symptoms such as convulsions.

TREATMENT

Agaricus muscarius 6c   In the early stages, associated with muscle twitchings and tremors, this remedy will prove useful. Dose: every two hours for four doses.

Strychninum 200c   This remedy is indicated to control a tendency to opisthotonus and will also help severe muscle twitching. Dose: four times daily for two days.

Gelsemium 200c   Muscular incoordination will be helped by the use of this remedy. It should also prevent paralytic symptoms appearing. Dose: three times daily for three days.

Opium 200c   Indicated when somnolent states arise, or signs of coma appear. Dose: every two hours for three doses.

13.   Lead Poisoning.   Chronic poisoning is occasionally met with, especially among animals grazing near factories, which use lead for processing, or those in the vicinity of lead mines.

SYMPTOMS

The recurrent laryngeal nerve shows paralysis leading to difficulty in inspiration. This may extend to the pharyngeal area, when difficulty in swallowing will be noticed, while paralysis of the lips is a common sequel. These signs accompany a dry skin, together with muscular weakness and stiffness.

TREATMENT

Gelsemium 200c   This remedy will probably be of most benefit in treating laryngeal and other paralyses of the head and throat. Dose: three times daily for four days. It may be necessary to prolong treatment with a lower potency, reducing the frequency of administration.

Cuprum metallicum 1M   Those cases showing muscular weakness and stiffness may be helped by Cuprum, more especially when there is muscular rigidity. Dose: once daily for seven days.

Curare 30c   Indicated in general muscular weakness, associated with excessive trembling of limbs. Dose: three times daily for three days.

Conium 200c   This remedy will be of especial benefit if the hind limbs show paralysis, symptoms gradually moving upwards and forwards. Dose: once daily for one week. It may be necessary to continue treatment with ascending potencies.

14.   Chronic Selenium Poisoning – Alkali Disease.   This may occur when there is a gradual intake of Selenium, by horses grazing on soils or pasture containing large amounts of selenium-rich plants.

SYMPTOMS
Emaciation, stiffness and lameness occur, together with loss of hair on the tail. Abnormality of the hooves occur, including coronitis leading to severe lameness.

TREATMENT

Cuprum metallicum 1M   This remedy will be of assistance when there is generalised muscle stiffness. Dose: once daily for seven days.

Arsenicum alb. 6c   This remedy will help control loss of hair along the base of the tail and will also promote appetite. Dose: night and morning for two weeks.

Calcarea fluorica 30c   When hoof abnormalities are prominent, this remedy will be of value. Dose: once daily for three weeks.

XXII Diseases of Unknown Etiology

1. **Post-Vaccinal Hepatitis.** This condition has been recorded as a sequel to infectious encephalomyelitis and may occur up to three months after contraction of the disease. It is usually related to the use of serum and vaccine used in controlling the disease, but some cases can arise independently. It has been reported in mares vaccinated against virus abortion and also in horses vaccinated against other diseases.

SYMPTOMS
The chief symptom is severe jaundice. Oliguria is present and nervous symptoms appear also. The head is pressed against any convenient object and the gait becomes incoordinated.

TREATMENT
Phosphorus 30c   Faeces pale. Petechial haemorrhage may occur on visible mucous membranes. Dose: three times daily for three days.

Chelidonium 30c   Yellow discolouration of the conjunctiva and visible mucous membranes. Possible tenderness over right shoulder region. Dose: three times daily for three days.

Carduus marianus 30c   Tenderness over liver region, with yellow stools. Dose: three times daily for four days.

Chionanthus 6x   Head symptoms. Conjunctiva yellow; stools yellow. Urine dark. Dose: three times daily for seven days.

Lycopodium 200c   Oliguria prominent. Urine contains sediment, reddish, and there may be abdominal distension. Dose: night and morning for one week.

Mercurius dulcis 6c   Bloated abdomen. Stools slimy, possibly blood-stained. Dose: night and morning for five days.

2.   **Grass Sickness.**   This is a non-infectious disease characterised by paralytic involvement of the nerve endings of the alimentary tract. It produces emaciation and extreme bowel stasis.
The age group commonly affected is three to six years and foals
do not contract the disease. While an occasional case has been
recorded in stabled animals, the great majority occur at pasture
in the early summer months.

SYMPTOMS
Acute, sub-acute and chronic types occur. In the acute form,
initial signs are anorexia and inability to swallow water. Bowel
movements cease and slight tympany is present, together with
frequent urination. Patchy sweating occurs and fine muscle
tremors are seen especially over the shoulder region. Stomach
contents run from the nose and frequently there is difficulty in
rising, the animal assuming a 'sitting-dog' posture. Rapid, wiry
pulse and brick-red discolouration of conjunctiva are indicative
of severe systemic disturbance. Sub-acute cases show a gaunt
'herring-gut' appearance and wasting of gluteal and femoral
muscles. Extreme restlessness causes the animal to pace round
the field in an aimless manner, and he may dip his head
frequently into a water trough in an attempt to drink. Bowel
stasis is not quite so severe in the sub-acute form, small quantities
of soft faeces being passed infrequently. This form may show a
temporary improvement, but soon lapses into a chronic form
characterised by intermittent bouts of abdominal pain, sweating
and excessive muscular weakness. Such cases invariably degenera-
te and if they are allowed to survive show acute symptoms the
following year.

TREATMENT
No effective treatment has yet been devised, probably because
there are no prodromal signs indicating disease. Once symptoms
appear, they worsen very rapidly and are invariably terminal.
Opportunities for studying and treating this disease are much
fewer than formerly when there were more susceptible animals
of the draught type to be found. The following remedies are
worthy of consideration and trial:—
Gelsemium 1M   In this high potency, it may be possible to
   influence favourably the paralytic involvement of the throat
   and mouth.

Plumbum metallicum Generalised paralysis, especially of the gut, can be helped by this remedy.

Conium When hind-leg paralysis occurs as in the 'sitting-dog' posture, this remedy may have great value.

Zincum metallicum Useful in controlling muscle tremors and patchy sweating.

Cocculus Associated lower limb paralysis and abdominal tympany.

Nux vomica This remedy may have some influence in helping bowel stasis especially in restlessness.

Lathyrus sativa The provings of this remedy suggest that it may be of value in restoring nerve function, if not completely lost.

Thallium Paralysis associated with this remedy extends to the lower abdomen and as such it may be of use in helping bowel stasis.

3. Colitis – Rudiosa Disease. This little known disease has assumed importance in the last decade or so. It takes the form of acute enteritis of the large bowel and affects mainly the adult animal.

SYMPTOMS
The inflammation is of very sudden onset and early signs are depression and discolouration of the conjunctivae. The pulse is very fast and thready and there is patchy sweating. Restlessness occurs with evidence of bowel pain, such as kicking at belly and looking round at the flanks. Foul smelling diarrhoea may occur but is not a constant symptom as the disease may be per-acute and leave no time for such a development. Dehydration occurs in less acute cases. The lesion in the caecum and colon is one of necrotic enteritis with haemorrhagic infiltration. The contents of the large bowel are fluid and foul smelling.

TREATMENT
In the less acute cases, which give room for medication, the following remedies should be tried: –

Arsenicum alb. 1M Give every hour for four or five doses.

Arnica 30c Passage of bright red blood accompanied by colic. Dose: every hour for four doses.

Baptisia 200c Tympanitic signs, especially on right side. There may be considerable flatus. Stools dark and watery. Dose: three times daily for three days.

Mercurius corrosivus 200c   Slimy mucus in stool, along with blood-stained lining of gut. Symptoms worse during the night. Severe colicky signs also present. Dose: every two hours for four doses.

4.   Thoroughbred Foal Disease.   This condition, occurring only in thoroughbred studs, is sometimes associated with too early curring of the umbilical cord with consequent interference with blood supply to the foal from the dam's placenta.

SYMPTOMS
Early signs are convulsions and paddling movements of the limbs. Recovery from this stage may lead into other stages showing different nervous symptoms. The disease commences during the first twenty-four hours. Weakness and aimless movements are accompanied by blindness. Nystagmus and sweating are prominent signs during convulsions and the foal may injure itself by striking the head on the floor. A comatose stage may supervene after which the animal passes into a stage in which reflexes are lost and blindness persists. In this stage the foal can walk, but blindness causes aimless wandering movements.

TREATMENT
Agaricus muscarius 6c   Give at the first suspicion of the disease developing. Dose: one hourly for five doses.
Belladonna 1M   Convulsions occur and the foal may strike the head on the ground. Dose: one hourly for five doses.
Stramonium 1M   Useful if nystagmus is a prominent symptom, also when aimless wandering occurs. Dose: one dose every two hours for four doses.
Opium 200c   For the comatose stage. Animal usually lies perfectly still. Dose: two doses four hours apart.
Hyoscyamus 200c   When blindness supervenes and early nervous signs appear, such as head shaking and early aimless movements. Dose: Two doses three hours apart.

5.   Enzootic Ataxia.   This disease affects young horses, principally thoroughbreds and saddle horses. The onset of the disease may have its origin in a fall or in some violent activity.

SYMPTOMS

Incoordination of movement is the first sign and in mild cases may not be noticeable unless the animal is ridden or exercised. Pressure over the cervical vertebrae causes pain. Knuckling occurs if the animal is pulled up sharply. Swaying of the hind-quarters is common. Intermittent dragging of feet and a disinclination to move or rise are seen in many cases. It is thought that symptoms are produced by compression of the spinal cord and this view is reinforced by the post-mortem finding of projections of vertebrae into the spinal canal. Inflammation of the articular processes of the thoracic and cervical vertebrae may be present.

TREATMENT

Conium 30c Weakness and incoordination of hind-limbs. Difficulty in rising. Dose: three times daily for three days.

Gelsemium 200c Knuckling and tendency to recumbency. Dose: three times daily for three days.

Lathyrus sativa 30c Spastic movements accompany rigidity of muscles. Difficulty in straightening up. Dose: three times daily for four days.

Agaricus muscarius 6c Pain over back, with tottering gait. Dose: three times daily for three days.

6. Sporadic Lymphangitis. This disease is characterised by fever lymphangitis and swelling of one or both hind legs.

SYMPTOMS

Febrile signs usher in the disease accompanied by rapid pulse and increased respiration. Pain is obvious and palpation of the area is resented. The limb is swollen and hot and may be carried off the ground. The lymphatics on the inside of the leg become thickened and the associated lymph glands become enlarged. The disease may persist for many weeks, producing a fibrous thickening of the limb. It frequently appears in animals fed on nutritious rations with little exercise. It can also be associated with superficial wounds which allow infection to gain access to underlying tissues. The resultant lymphadenitis causes in turn a septic lymphangitis.

TREATMENT

Aconitum napellus 6c   Always give first, in the early febrile
stage. Dose: every hour for four doses.

Calcarea fluorica 30c   Early inflammation of the lymphatics and
later fibrous stage. Dose: three times daily for four days.

Kali bichromicum 30c   Serum oozes from the inflamed lymphatics. Dose: three times daily for three days.

Apis 6c   Oedema accompanies lymphangitis. Dose: every two
hours for four doses.

Rhus toxicodendrom 30c   Superficial skin lesions become inflamed and erysipelatous. Dose: three times daily for three
days.

Externally, a lotion of *Rhus toxicodendron* and *Arnica* will be
helpful.

7.   **Anhydrosis.**   This condition is characterised by the absence
of sweating and occurs mainly in humid climates among horses
imported from more temperate zones.

SYMPTOMS

Although excessive sweating occurs in the early stages, this soon
disappears and any sweating appearing later is patchy in distribution and confined to the skin under the the mane. Skin becomes
dry and scaly. Acute pyrexia occurs and dyspnoea becomes
severe. The temperature may rise as high as 108° F.

TREATMENT

Aconitum napellus 6c   Early in acute febrile stage. Dose: hourly
for four doses.

Arsenicum alb. 1M   Skin dry and scaly. Dose: three times daily
for three days.

Arsenicum iodatum 6c   Respiratory signs. Dyspnoea. Dose:
every three hours for four doses.

Calcarea carbonica 200c   Patchy sweating. Dose: one dose per
day for four days.

Alumina 30c   Excessive dryness of skin, with itching. Tendency
to constipation. Dose: night and morning for four days.

Berberis aquifolium 6c   This remedy will promote glandular
activity and help promote sweating. Dose: three times daily
for ten days.

Petroleum 6c   Dry, scaly skin, with pyrexia. Remedy stimulates sweat glands. Dose: three times daily for five days.

Nux moschata 6c   Extreme dryness of skin accompanied by weakness and faltering gait. Dose: three times daily for five days.

XXIII Metabolic Diseases

1. **Lactation Tetany of Mares – Eclampsia.** This condition is
accompanied by hypo-calcaemia, and in cases which have a
history of recent transportation, by a hypo-magnesaemia also.
It occurs usually about the tenth day after foaling, or again a
few days after weaning. It is commonest in mares which are
lactating heavily and may be brought on by hard physical work,
or prolonged transport. Mares requiring medicinal help at the
foaling heat are usually more severely affected than those
showing symptoms following transportation.

SYMPTOMS
Profuse sweating occurs and movement becomes difficult because
of tetanic spasm of the muscle of the limbs. Respiration becomes
difficult and dilation of nostrils is evident. Tremors of the jaw
and shoulder muscles occur, but there is no aversion to light
(unlike tetanus). The pulse becomes rapid and irregular. Cessation of urination and bowel movements are common sequelae.
In the later stages convulsions appear and may become continuous. Recovery is associated with large quantities of urine.

TREATMENT
To supplement the use of normal calcium injections, which
normally promote recovery, the following remedies will help to
minimise the risk of damage to the central nervous system and
prevent relapse.
Calcarea carbonica 200c   This remedy is especially suitable for
    fat mares which show abundant sweating. Dose: every hour
    for four doses.
Magnesium phosphoricum 6c   This remedy can be used in
    alternation with the previous one, for cases associated with
    hypomagnesaemia. Dose: every hour for four doses.
Cuprum metallicum 6c   This remedy will be useful in controll-

ing muscle cramps, associated with rigidity. Dose: every two hours for four doses.

Belladonna 1M   Indicated in those cases showing convulsions. The patient is excitable prior to the onset of symptoms. The pupils become dilated, there is head shaking and a full bounding pulse. Dose: every hour for four doses.

Agaricus muscarius 6c   When this remedy is called for, the animal tends to fall backwards or sideways. If given early enough it may prevent convulsions. Dose: every two hours for four doses.

2.   Paralytic Myoglobinuria – Azoturia.   This disease occurs during exercise and appears after a period of rest, during which time the animal has been receiving full rations. Muscular degeneration is the main feature of the condition, associated with myoglobinuria – the appearance in the urine of muscle pigment. In the majority of cases there is complete inactivity for two or more days before exercise. A rest of twenty-four hours or more than two weeks is unlikely to produce the condition. Attacks may occur after general anaesthesia and it has been reported in horses grazing good pasture land for a few days and then subjected to hard work. It is thought that a lack of vitamin E may be a contributory cause.

SYMPTOMS

The gluteal muscles are most frequently affected and become hard and painful. The affected muscles liberate myoglobin, which subsequently appears in the urine, colouring it dark reddish brown. Sweating appears as the first sign which comes on about one hour after exercise has started. The animal becomes averse to movement but if made to move, shows stiffness of gait. Recumbency soon sets in, pain and restlessness are evident and there is an increase in respiration. The pulse is hard and wiry and the temperature is raised. Both hind legs are invariably affected, the muscles of the upper region becoming hard and board-like. Less severe cases show slight lameness and tenderness over the sacral region, with restricted movement.

TREATMENT

Aconitum napellus 6c   Should always be given as early as possible in the febrile stage. Dose: hourly for four doses.

Belladonna 1M   Indicated when there are signs of nervousness, dilated pupils, full bounding pulse and a smooth, hot skin. Dose: hourly for four doses.

Thallium 30c   This remedy may be of use in the early paralytic stage, accompanied by sweating. Dose: three times daily for three days.

Berberis vulgaris 30c   When there is pain and tenderness over the kidney region with pronounced stiffness, this remedy is indicated. Dose: three times daily for three days.

Arnica 30c   This is a good, general remedy indicated at the commencement of symptoms in most cases. It may be associated with a fear of being approached or touched. Dose: two doses three hours apart.

Bryonia 30c   Indicated when stiffness or tenseness of muscles is associated with disinclination to move. The animal is better at rest. Dose: three times daily for two days.

Rhus toxicodendron 1M   When this remedy is needed, the symptoms are ameliorated when the animal can be made to move. There is heat and tenderness over the sacral region. Dose: every two hours for four doses.

Bellis perennis 30c   This is a principle remedy. There is congestion of local blood vessels and it is also associated with unduly dark urine. Dose: three times daily for two days.

Cimicifuga 30c   Indicated when there is twitching of muscles, accompanied by stiffness and restlessness. Dose: three times daily for three days.

Helonias 30c   This is a useful remedy in mild cases, especially indicated when mares are affected. Dose: three times daily for three days.

XXIV Fore Leg Lameness

1.   **Inflammation of Bicipital Bursa – Bicipital Bursitis.**   This bursa is found between the tendon of the biceps brachii muscle and the bicipital groove of the humerus. The bursa together with its tendon may become the seat of inflammation which may be either acute or chronic. It frequently arises as a result of a blow to the point of the shoulder. An infective bursitis can arise from streptococcal diseases and from brucellosis.

SYMPTOMS
The horse tries to advance the limb without flexion and this causes lifting of the head. Consequent on poor flexion, the foot is lifted from the ground with difficulty. On moving forward, there is a shortened stride and stumbling occurs. The shoulder joint (scapulo humeral) becomes fixed and is one of the major signs of shoulder lameness. The limb may be moved in an outward circular fashion in an attempt to move forward without advancing the limb. The leg may be carried in acute cases. At rest the affected limb is drawn slightly backwards and the animal rests on the toe.

TREATMENT
Ruta graueolens 6c   Flexor muscles and tendons are injured. There may also be additional periostitis. Dose: three times daily for three days.
Arnica 30c   Always give this remedy as a routine measure. Dose: one dose twelve hours apart for two doses.
Apis 6c   Synovitis of the bursa. Dose: every two hours for four doses.
Benzoic Acid 6c   Accompanying nephritis yielding offensive urine. Dose: two hourly for three doses.
Bryonia 6c   Animal is relieved by pressure over the bursa region and symptoms worse on movement. Dose: three times daily for three days.

Kali muriaticum 30c   Joint swelling, involving surrounding areas. Worse in warm conditions. Dose: three times daily for three days.

Hypericum 1M   Damage to nerve endings. Dose: once daily for two days.

2.   Radial Paralysis.   The radial nerve supplies impulses to the elbow, knee and digital joints, together with the ulnaris lateralis muscle — the lateral flexor of the carpal or knee joint. Paralysis of varying degrees arises usually from some injury at the point where the nerve crosses the musculo-spiral groove of the humerus. This could happen from a kick at this point, or from a fall.

SYMPTOMS
These vary according to the degree of nerve damage. If the extensor tendons of the digit are affected the animal is unable to advance the limb. Dropped elbow is apparent when the branch of the nerve supplying the triceps muscle is involved and this also causes flexion of the digits. This makes the limb appear longer than usual. Mild cases may show little more than stumbling or slight lameness when walking slowly.

TREATMENT
Gelsemium 200c   Stumbling and weakness of leg muscles. Dose: three times daily for three days.

Plumbum metallicum 6c   Extensor tendons show involvement and reflexes are diminished. Dose: three times daily for four days.

Curare 30c   Weakness of muscles is associated with trembling and loss of reflex action. Dose: three times daily for five days.

Ruta graueolens 6c   Tendon injury, with possible periostitis. Dose: night and morning for one week.

Arnica 30c   Paralysis resulting from kick or fall. Dose: every twelve hours for two doses.

3.   Hygroma of Carpus or Knee.   This is a synovial swelling affecting the bursa of the knee joint on its anterior surface. The tendon sheaths of the associated extensor muscles may also be involved. It is caused by injury and can exist as a result of the animal repeatedly striking the knee against a manger or stall.

SYMPTOMS

A swelling occurs over the knee joint, the swelling containing synovial fluid. There may be additional swellings in the joint region depending on which tissues are involved. Acute cases show pain on pressure while neglected cases show fibrous thickening.

TREATMENT

Apis 6c   Acute cases showing tenderness and oedema of the joint, with synovial effusion. Dose: every two hours for four doses.

Bryonia 6c   Joint hard, shiny and tense. Pressure on joint relieves pain. Worse on movement. Dose: three times daily for four days.

Ruta graveolens 30c   Associated tendon sheaths are involved. Dose: night and morning for four days.

Silicea 200c   Fibrous tissue develops in neglected cases. Dose: once daily for two weeks.

Calcarea fluorica 30c   Chronic synovitis with lumpy deposits showing in joint. Dose: once daily for ten days.

Hepar sulphuris 200c   Hygroma infected with pyogenic bacteria. Dose: night and morning for one week.

4.   Carpitis.   This is acute or chronic inflammation of the knee joint and may involve the joint capsule and associated ligaments. Early movement is an arthritis which, if neglected, can lead to more severe osteoarthritis. The main cause is an injury such as concussion to the joint and is frequently seen in animals subjected to hard exercise.

SYMPTOMS

The anterior surface of the knee bones becomes the seat of pathological change, along with the distal end of the radius and may involve bony structures as far down as the third metacarpal bone. Changes bring about the deposition of new bone as a consequence of periostitis. Osteoarthritis develops in those cases which involve bone change. Mild arthritis develops in those cases where no body changes take place. Lameness may not be evident in chronic cases, although enlargements are evident over the area, either fibrous or bony.

TREATMENT

Ruta graueolens 30c   Accompanying periostitis. Dose: three times daily for three days.

Rhus toxicodendron 1M   Mild arthritis, when animal shows improvement on exercise. Dose: once daily for one week.

Calcarea fluorica 30c   Bony exostoses develop. Dose: night and morning for three days, followed by one dose daily for three weeks.

Silicea 200c   Fibrous enlargements in chronic cases. Dose: once daily for ten days.

Hekla lava 12c   A useful remedy for bony exostoses. Dose: one twice daily for one week.

5.   Contraction of Superficial Digital Flexor – The Perforatus Tendon.   Contraction of this tendon may be congenital or acquired. If the former, the condition is usually present in both limbs; if the latter, it is normally unilateral.

SYMPTOMS

Knuckling of fetlocks is one early sign. Severe contraction may lead to the animal walking on the front part of the fetlock.

TREATMENT

In the young animal, if the contraction is not so severe as to warrant surgical correction, the following remedies will be of use: –

Ruta graveolens 6c   Periosteum affected, a likely sequel if the condition is acquired due to an injury. Dose: three times daily for one week.

Rhus Toxicodendron 1M   Contraction accompanied by heat and tenderness. Improvement with exercise. Dose: night and morning for four days.

Arnica 30c   Condition associated with injury and shock. Dose: every twelve hours for two doses.

Externally, the application of a lotion of *Arnica* and *Ruta* is beneficial.

6.   Tendinitis – Tenosynovitis.   This is the name given to inflammation of one or both of the flexor tendons, the perforans (deep) and the perforatus (superficial) and their associated tendon sheaths. The injury which produces this condition causes a tearing of the sheath attachments from their insertion on the tendons. This causes inflammation and transient slight haemorrhage. This in turn produces adhesions between the tendons and also between tendons and sheath, leading to formation of fibrous or scar tissue.

SYMPTOMS
The tendons assume a bowed appearance resulting from adhesions developing on the volar (posterior) aspect of the metacarpal region. There are various names for this condition: (a) High Tendovaginitis, involving the area immediately below the carpus, (b) Middle Tendovaginitis, involving the middle third of the metacarpus or cannon, and (c) Low Tendovaginitis, the area involving the volar annular ligament and the distal third of the cannon bone.

While the condition may be seen in the high or low areas alone, the middle area involves one of the other two. High and middle involvement is commoner in the fore leg and arises as a result of severe strain of the flexor area. Low area involvement is the rule when the hind limb is affected. Early symptoms include sudden lameness after severe exercise, producing a diffuse swelling of the affected area, with pain on palpation. There is pointing of the toe to ease pressure on the heel area and the animal favours the toe when made to move. When the condition becomes chronic it is evidenced by a firm, fibrous swelling over the flexor area. Such animals may not show lameness unless subjected to severe exercise.

TREATMENT
Arnica 30c   Should be given as soon as possible after injury sustained. Dose: every twelve hours for two doses.
Ruta graveolens 30c   Severe cases, with haemorrhage and consequent threat of periostitis. Dose: three hourly for four doses.
Rhus toxicodendron 1M   Tendon inflammation generally. Pain eased by movement. Dose: night and morning for four days.
Apis 6c   Oedematous swellings, especially over fetlock area. Swellings usually hot and puffy. Dose: two hourly for five doses.
Silicea 200c   Chronic cases. This remedy will help resorption of fibrous tissue. Dose: once daily for ten days.
Externally, the application of *Arnica* and *Rhus* liniments will be of benefit.

7. Metacarpal Periostitis — Sore Shins.   This is a periostititis of the anterior surface of the third metacarpal bone. It is of comparatively rare occurrence in the hind limb, but common in the fore limbs of young racing animals. Concussion is the predisposing cause and both fore limbs may be simultaneously involved. Injuries to the periosteum from blows may also account for some cases.

SYMPTOMS

The main sign is a painful swelling on the anterior surface of the metacarpal bone and is warm to the touch. Subcutaneous oedema may be present. Lameness is increased on exercise and the step becomes shortened. Shifting from one limb to the other occurs in bilateral involvement.

TREATMENT

Arnica 30c   Always begin treatment with two doses, twelve hours apart.

Ruta graveolens 6c   This is one of the main remedies. Will prevent formation of exostosis. Dose: three times daily for three days.

Apis 6c   Oedema prominent under the skin. Dose: two hourly for four doses.

Calcarea fluorica 30c   Neglected cases, if deposits have started on the bone. Dose: once daily for ten days.

Externally, the affected area should be bathed with *Ruta* and *Arnica* lotions.

8.   Splints.   The fore limbs are usually affected in this condition of young horses. The lesion to which the name 'splints' has been applied is found on the inner aspect of the limb between the second and third metacarpal bones. The interosseous ligament between these bones is the seat of the trouble, injury to the periosteum causing the formation of new bone growth. The metatarsal bones are less commonly affected. Injuries by blows may cause the condition, but the chief cause is concussion due to hard work or exercise. The condition is most ocmmon in the two year age group.

SYMPTOMS

Lameness seen especially when the animal trots is an early sign.

Swelling, accompanied by heat and pain are soon evident. The usual site of splints is about three inches below the knee on the inside of the leg. There may be one large swelling, or two or three small swellings. Once the swelling subsides it becomes firmer due to deposition of new bone.

TREATMENT

Arnica 30c   Give as early as possible once the injury has been sustained. Dose: two doses twelve hours apart.

Ruta graveolens 6c   Will help control periostitis and prevent exostosis. Dose: three times daily for three days.

Silicea 200c   Exostosis develop in neglected case. Dose: once daily for ten days.

Calcarea fluorica 30c   Exostosis in region of small carpal bones. Dose: once daily for ten days.

Externally, an application of *Ruta* and *Arnica* liniments will be of benefit.

9.   **Sprain of the Suspensory Ligament.**   This ligament is the main support tendon of the leg below the knee and sprain of this structure is usually confined to the forelimb. It is invariably produced by an injury. Extreme extension of the fetlock joint can put a heavy strain on the ligament at the point of bifurcation in the lower third of the metacarpal area. It is most likely to occur at the end of a period of long exercise or a hard race. Periostitis may arise if the ligament becomes injured at its attachment to the sesamoid bones, causing formation of new growth.

SYMPTOMS

Lameness is acute and usually involves the flexor tendons as well as the ligament. Swelling is the first sign, with the heel resting on the ground. The fetlock joint is held in an extensor fashion. Chronic involvement of the ligament produces fibrous swelling usually at the point of bifurcation. Palpation of the limb in the region of the sesamoid bones will reveal if any injury has occurred. Thickening of the area will indicate this, and also in the distal metacarpal third where bifurcation occurs.

TREATMENT

Arnica 30c   Give immediately sprain has occurred. Dose: two doses twelve hours apart.

Rhus toxicodendron 1M   This remedy will help reduce inflammation and extend its action to tendons as well as ligament. Dose: three times daily for two days.

Ruta graveolens 200c   Periostitis in region of sesamoid bones. Dose: twice daily for four days.

Silicea 30c   In chronic sprain will aid resorption of fibrous thickening. Dose: once daily for ten days.

Externally, the application of *Rhus, Ruta* and *Arnica* liniment will assist greatly.

10.   Sesamoiditis.   This is an inflammation of the sesamoid bones at the bottom of the metacarpal bone. It produces periostitis and deposition of new bone growth. It is due to abnormally heavy strain on the fetlock area.

SYMPTOMS

Pain and swelling are first noticed on the volar aspect of the fetlock joint and the area is extremely sensitive to pressure. The fetlock is held in an abnormal position to avoid pressure being put on it. Bony changes will appear about three weeks after the initial injury.

TREATMENT

Arnica 30c   Give as soon as possible after injury has been sustained. Dose: every three hours for two doses.

Ruta graveolens 200c   This will hasten resolution of periostitis and help prevent formation of new bone growth. Dose: twice daily for four days.

Calc fluorica 30c   Neglected cases where exostosis has already occurred. Dose: once a week for four weeks.

Silicea 30c   This will help remove fibrous tissue in chronic cases. Dose: once daily for ten days.

Externally, the application of *Ruta* and *Arnica* lotions will be beneficial.

11.   Periostitis of the Fetlock Joint.   Inflammation occurring at the distal end of the metacarpal bone and the proximal end of the first phalanx produces this condition. Mild cases show no more than a simple arthritis without formation of new bone. It is commonest in the fore limbs. The two year age group of racing animals is most commonly affected. Concussion is the main cause and bad conformation of the pastern predisposes to it. The lateral digital extensor is frequently implicated and the resulting periostitis produces new growth which may or may not involve the articular surfaces.

SYMPTOMS
The joint capsule of the fetlock joint is distended on the volar (posterior) surface underneath the suspensory ligament. Osteo-arthritis supervenes if the joint is implicated in deposition of new growth. Palpation of the limb produces pain in the area and swelling is evident. Fibrous thickening of tissue on the anterior surfaces can be seen. The animal may point the toe and if made to exercise, the lameness gets worse.

TREATMENT
Arnica 30c   Give first for the initial injury. Dose: two doses, three hours apart.
Ruta graveolens 200c   This will aid considerably in overcoming the condition and will help control deposition of new bone. Dose: twice daily for four days.
Apis 30c   Inflammatory fluid gathers in the joint apsule. Dose: every hour for four doses.
Silicea 30c   In chronic cases, this will help resorption of fibrous tissue. Dose: once daily for ten days.
Calcarea fluorica 30c   When exostoses have already occurred. Dose: once a week for four weeks.
Bryonia 200c   Heat and tenderness occur in early stages. A guiding symptom for its use; worse on movement or better by pressure. Dose: every two hours for four doses.

12.   **Ringbone – Phalangeal Exostoses.**   This term implies new bone growth occurring on one or other of the phalanges resulting from a periostitis. It leads to ankylosis of the pastern or coffin joint, dependent on an osteoarthritis. There are two varieties:—
(1) High Ringbone in which the distal end of the first and the proximal end of the second phalanx become involved in new bone growth.
(2) Low Ringbone in which new bone growth involves the distal end of the second phalanx and the proximal end of the third.
   Ringbone may be articular when new bone growth involves

the joint surfaces, or periarticular when confined to the area surrounding them. The latter is common in high ringbone. The primary cause is concussion producing a periostitis resulting from the injury caused by pulling or detachment of associated ligaments. Ringbone is more common in the fore-limb.

SYMPTOMS
Heat and swelling occur initially and lameness is evident. In low ringbone there may be a stiffening of the hair over the coronary band. Periarticular ringbone may show no lameness but the swelling will be obvious.

TREATMENT
Arnica 30c   Give as early as possible after injury. Dose: two doses three hours apart.
Ruta graveolens 200c   Will help control periostitis if given early. Dose: night and morning for four days.
Calc fluorica 30c   Tendency to develop exostoses. Dose: once weekly for four weeks.
Silicea 30c   Developing fibrosis. Dose: once daily for two weeks.
Externally, a liniment of *Ruta* and *Arnica* will help in the early stages.

13.   Pyramidal Disease.   When the exterior process of the third phalanx is involved in deposition of new bone growth, it is given this name. It is usually due to an underlying periostitis. The digital extensor tendon is frequently involved in the cause of the disease, when it is subjected to excessive strain at its attachment to the extensor process of the third phalanx. Deposition of new bone is the result in the form of a large callus.

SYMPTOMS
The centre area of the hoof shows a swelling at the coronary band. The animal may point the toe of the affected limb. Heat, pain and swelling are early signs and lameness is evident. Osteoarthritis at the coffin joint follows when the condition becomes chronic.

TREATMENT
The same remedies apply here as for Ringbone, but Calc. fluor. is a principle remedy.

4. Quittor. This is a chronic inflammation of the lateral cartilages leading to necrosis and the formation of a purulent sinus. The forelimbs are more commonly affected. Abscess under the coronary band due to injury may cause the condition as may any injury introducing infection to the area of the cartilage.

SYMPTOMS
Either cartilage may be involved and the condition commences as an inflammatory lesion of the coronary band above the cartilage. Sinus formation occurs, discharging purulent material. Lameness is common only in the acute stage.

TREATMENT
Arnica 30c   If injury suspected. Dose: Two doses three hours apart.
Hypericum 1M   Early stages, if ragged or punctured wounds are involved. Dose: two hourly for three doses.
Ledum 6c   Symptoms similar to those of Hypericum. Dose: two hourly for four doses.
Hepar sulphuris 6x or 200c   In the acute, tender, inflammatory stage, this will promote quick healing. Given in high potency at this stage it will prevent suppuration. Once pus has gathered, low potency will hasten its elimination. Dose 6x: every hour for four doses. 200c: three times daily for two days.
Silicea 30c   Once a sinus has developed in an established case this remedy will help removal of necrotic tissue, leading to healthy granulation. Dose: once daily for one week.
Externally, a lotion of *Calendula* will effect quick healing in stubborn cases.

15. Sidebones. This term implies ossification of the lateral cartilages usually in the forefeet. It is probably caused by concussion in the region of the quarter of the wall producing a primary inflammation of the lateral cartilage.

SYMPTOMS
Pain is evident if palpation is exerted during the process of bone deposition. In the established case the cartilage loses its normal resilient feel and bone formation can be felt. Lameness is not always present but when it does occur it is usually related to the inflammatory stage.

TREATMENT
This is essentially the same as for Ringbone and Pyramidal Disease.

16.   Laminitis.   This is an inflammation of the sensitive laminae of the foot leading to an acute local congestion. The pressure of this blood on the laminae causes severe pain. Acute and chronic forms of the condition are recognised and may involve two front or two hind feet or all four together. The fore feet are more commonly affected. Predisposing causes may be systemic or may be due to bacterial infection.

SYMPTOMS
(1) The acute form: — When the fore feet are involved, the animal assumes a position where the hind-feet are drawn under the body to relieve pressure on the fore feet which are extended, the heels taking the weight of the animal. There is great disinclination to move and the feet can be raised only with difficulty. External signs include heat over the coronary band and the wall. The digital arteries show a bounding pulse and the animal exhibits acute pain, anxious expression, sweating and increased respiration. The conjunctiva become brick-coloured. In parturient laminitis as a result of metritis due to retention of infected placenta, there is usually a rise of temperature sometimes as high as 107° F and a discharge of blood-stained fluid from the uterus.
(2) The chronic form: — Displacement of the third phalanx takes place due to separation of sensitive and insensitive laminae, resulting in rotation of the phalanx. This displacement is usually permanent. The sole becomes flat and when the animal moves, the heel is put to the ground in an exaggerated manner. The wall of the heel grows more rapidly than usual and shows as rings on the wall surface, dependent on inflammation of the coronary band. Mild or sub-acute attacks may occur during the chronic stage if predisposing conditions such as rich grazing arise.

TREATMENT
Aconitum napellus 30c   This should be given immediately the first symptoms are seen, and will help to allay anxiety and regulate pulse and respiration. Dose: every 30 mins. for six doses.

Belladonna 1M   Throbbing arteries, full bounding pulse, pyrexia and sweating. Dose: every 30 mins. for six doses. Aconite and Belladonna may be given together in the same dosage.

Nux vomica 1M   Systemic congestion. Dose: every two hours for four doses.

Calc fluorica 30c   Tissue involvement in the chronic case. This remedy will help reduce involvement and promote a return to normal structure if not too far advanced. Dose: once a week for four weeks.

17.   Seedy Toe.   This is a complication of chronic laminitis due to separation of sensitive and insensitive laminae allowing infection to gain entrance to the sensitive laminae. This causes a purulent discharge from the white line.

TREATMENT

Silicea 30c   This is the main remedy in controlling septic involvement. Dose: once daily for one week.

Hepar sulphuris 6c   This should be used in the early acute stage. Dose: hourly for four doses.

Externally bathing with *Calendula* lotion will assist healing.

18.   Navicular Disease.   This is a bursitis of the perforans tendon bursa where it joins the navicular bone, causing adhesions between the bone and the deep flexor tendon. The inflammation set up may lead to decalcification of the bone itself. The condition is confined to the fore feet. Concussion is thought to play a part in its development and it is particularly liable to occur in horses put to heavy work on hard ground. Pressure is put on the bone where the deep flexor tendon attaches and this is thought to be instrumental in producing bursitis. There is frequently a history of intermittent lameness which improves on resting. Both fore feet may be involved but the lameness is usually worse in one than in the other. Brucellosis has been thought to be a contributory cause.

SYMPTOMS

These may disappear at rest, but always re-appear on exercise. Pointing of the toe is common and this may be seen alternately if both feet are involved. During movement the toe takes the weight of the animal, most noticeable when walking or trotting.

The toe may show excessive wear. Pressure over the frog evinces pain and this is increased when the animal is turned in the direction of the affected foot. In prolonged affections, the foot changes shape, due to lack of pressure on the frog. The heels become contracted and the foot assumes a "box-like" appearance. The concavity of the sole is accentuated and the foot becomes elongated. Changes occurring in the navicular bone itself include necrosis and osteo porosis and fibrous adhesions develop in the bursa.

TREATMENT

Bryonia 200c   Early acute inflammatory stage. Dose: every hour for four doses.

Ruta graveolens 200c   Periostitis present. Dose: twice daily for three days.

Apis 30c   Synovitis suspected, with oedematous effusion. Dose: hourly for four doses.

Calcarea fluorica 30c   Established cases. This remedy will help control exostoses and bony changes. Dose: once a week for four weeks.

Silicea 200c   Fibrous adhesions develop in the bursa. Dose: once daily for five days.

Brucella abortus nosode 30c   This should be given as a routine along with other indicated remedies. Dose: once weekly for three weeks.

Hepar sulphuris 200c   Early acute inflammatory stage. This will also be beneficial in established bursitis if brucellosis is implicated. Dose: night and morning for two days.

19.   Corns.   These occur in the angle formed by the wall and the bar of the foot and include the sensitive and insensitive tissues of the foot. Corns usually occur on the fore feet and favour the inner angle. Any pressure on this area may produce a corn. Lack of frog pressure is also a predisposing cause. A history of laminitis may result in the development of a corn. Corns may be dry, moist or suppurating. The first is due to bruising of sensitive tissue causing haemorrhage, showing as a red stain in the corn area. Severe injury can lead to a moist corn with the appearance of serum underneath the injured sole and infection of this type leads to the suppurative form.

SYMPTOMS

Lameness varies according to location of the corn. The animal tends to put weight on the toe to decrease pressure over the affected area.

TREATMENT

Arnica 30c   Give this remedy first, as the corn usually develops form an injury. Dose: two doses three hours apart.

Calcarea fluorica 30c   This remedy will aid absorption of hard tissue and promote growth of healthy horn. Dose: once a week for four weeks.

Silicea 30c   In suppurative corns, this remedy will control infection and prevent necrosis of tissue. Dose: once daily for ten days.

XXV Lameness of the Hind Limb

1. **Iliac Thrombosis.**   Damage by strongyle worms may arise in the posterior aorta and the iliac artery, leading to an arteritis. The resulting thrombosis leads to circulatory interference causing lameness.

SYMPTOMS
Lameness usually supervenes after a short period of exercise and the severity depends on the size of the thrombus. Severe cases may show lameness when walking. Anxiety, pain and sweating accompany the lameness, but sweating is absent over the affected area. The affected limb loses some of its warm feeling. Lameness is intermittent, disappearing on rest and appearing again on exercise.

TREATMENT
Bothrops 30c   Condition accompanied by nervous trembling, with possible bowel haemorrhage. Dose: three hourly for three doses.
Lachesis 30c   Rectal straining, with pain over the sacral region. Dose: two hourly for four doses.
Calcarea fluorica 30c   This remedy will hasten dissolution of the thrombus and resolution of the aneurism. Dose: once a week for four weeks.
Vipera 6c   Associated cramping of muscles of the limb, with possibly an accompanying jaundice. Dose: three times daily for four days.

2. **Bursitis of the Tendon of the Middle Gluteus Muscle.**   This inflammation arises when the bursa is affected as the tendon passes over the great trochanter of the femur. Falling on this area or strain of the tendon can bring it about.

SYMPTOMS
Pain becomes evident over the great trochanter if pressure is
applied. Flexion of the limb is common at rest while weight is
placed on the inside of the foot when the animal moves. This
causes the inside wall to wear more than the outside and movement tends to go towards the sound limb.

TREATMENT
Apis 30c   Synovitis. Oedema of the Bursa. Dose: two hourly
   for four doses.
Bryonia 30c   Relief from pressure. Symptoms worse on movement. Dose: two hourly for four doses.
Ruta graveolens 200c   Tendency to periostitis. Dose: night and
   morning for three days.
Note:—   The possibility of infection by Brucella abortus as a
   cause should not be forgotten. The use of the nosode
   in treatment will help considerably if this is the case.

3.   **Crural Paralysis. Paralysis of Femoral Nerve.**   The quadri-
ceps group of muscles is involved in this paralysis being made up
of the rectus femoris, the vastus lateralis, the vastus medialis and
the vastus intermedius. It covers the area of the front of the
femur and both sides. Azoturia has been listed as a cause of this
paralysis which also arises from injury.

SYMPTOMS
When standing, all joints become flexed and no weight is put on
the leg. There is difficulty in advancing the limb.

TREATMENT
Arnica 30c   Always if injury is suspected. Two doses three hours
   apart.
Gelsemium 200c   Accompanying weakness and lassitude. Dose:
   night and morning for four days.
Conium 30c   Tendency for paralysis to ascend, affecting areas
   further up the limb. Dose: night and morning for one week.
Plumbum metallicum 30c   Difficulty in extending the limb.
   Reflexes are lost and the foot may be swollen. Dose: night
   and morning for one week.

4.   **Gonitis.**   This term is used to denote inflammation of the

stifle joint and leads to arthritis. It may be caused by injuries to the bones forming the joint and associated cartilages and ligaments. Infective agents can produce arthritis of this joint, e.g. navel-ill, brucellosis and E. coli infection.

SYMPTOMS
Lameness varies according to the severity of the injury. If the joint cartilages are involved, lameness can be severe. The joint capsule becomes swollen and hot and pain is evident when the animal moves the leg forward. Flexion of the limb is usual to avoid putting the foot on the ground as this aggravates the pain.

TREATMENT
Apis 30c   Inflammation is accompanied by oedema of the joint capsule. Dose: two hourly for four doses.
Bryonia 30c   Joint swollen, pressure relieves, symptoms worse on movement. Dose: two hourly for four doses.
Ruta graveolens 200c   Periostitis round the joint. Dose: night and morning for four days.
Rhus toxicodendron 1M   Arthritis of joint developing. Dose: once daily for one week.
Streptococcus Nosode 30c   Navel-ill infection suspected to have led to the condition. Dose: once daily for three days.
Brucella abortus nosode 30c   If brucellosis suspected, one dose daily for three days.

5.   **Stringhalt.**   This is an involuntary flexion of the hock during progression, affecting one or both hind limbs. The lateral digital extensor is usually involved, injury of some kind being considered the cause. Adhesions may form as the tendon crosses the lateral surface of the hock joint.

SYMPTOMS
These vary from mild flexion to a severe involuntary movement which brings the leg up almost to the abdomen. The condition is exaggerated when the animal is made to turn round sharply.

TREATMENT
Strychninum 200c   This remedy will help reduce the spasmodic flexion. Dose: once daily for five days.
Arnica 30c   Give at once if injury suspected. Dose: two doses

three hours apart.

Gelsemium 200c   Tendency to accompanying paralysis. Dose: once daily for five days.

6.   Bone Spavin.   This is a periostitis or osteitis affecting the inside of the hock joint below the articular surface of the main joint. It causes osteoarthritis and ankylosis of the tarsal joints. Poor conformation contributes to the condition and it can be precipitated by injuries.

SYMPTOMS

Pain is evident on flexion of the joint and there is a shortening of the forward movement. The animal always puts the toe on the ground first. Lameness is worse when the animal moves after rest and mild cases can improve on exercise. Severe flexion of the joint causes increased lameness when the animal is moved immediately afterwards.

TREATMENT

Rhus toxicodendron 1M   Cases which improve on exercise. Dose: once daily for one week.

Ruta graveolens 200c   Early stages, when periostitis first develops. Dose: three times daily for two days.

Arnica 30c   When injury is suspected as the contributing cause. Dose: Two doses three hours apart.

7.   Bog Spavin.   This term implies a swelling of the joint capsule with fluid seen on the antero-medial aspect of the hock joint. Injury to the hock joint can predispose to the condition which is characterised by three fluctuating swellings.

SYMPTOMS

The largest swelling is located at the antero-medial aspect of the hock joint. Two smaller swellings occur on either side of the posterior surface of the joint. Pressure on any one swelling causes an increase in the others. When due to injury there will be local heat and pain, and lameness occurs, but this is absent when the condition is due to other causes.

TREATMENT

Arnica 30c   Give at once if injury has occurred. Dose: two doses three hours apart.

Apis 30c   Oedema and synovitis. Give early in the inflammatory stage. It will also reduce fluid in non-inflammatory cases. Dose: once three times daily for three days.

Bryonia 30c   Helpful in inflammatory states where there is tenderness over the joint and pressure relieves. Dose: two hourly for four weeks.

8.   Curb.   This is an enlargement at the posterior aspect of the fibular-tarsal bone. It is dependent on inflammation and thickening of the plantar ligament. Poor conformation puts stress on the plantar ligament and this is a predisposing cause. Violent exertion can also cause curb.

SYMPTOMS

The condition is characterised by an enlargement on the posterior surface of the fibular-tarsal bone. Inflammation and lameness are present in the acute phase. The heel becomes elevated and swelling appears over the area which does not decrease on exercise. In chronic cases, tissues surrounding the area may become infiltrated with scar tissue.

TREATMENT

Arnica 30c   Condition due to violent exercise, concussion or injury. Dose: two doses three hours apart.

Rhus toxicodendron 1M   Acute inflammatory stage, especially if there is improvement on exercise. Dose: two hourly for four doses.

Ruta graveolens 200c   Periostitis. This remedy will help prevent deposition of new bone. Dose: night and morning for three days.

Silicea 200c   In chronic cases, this remedy will hasten absorption of scar tissue. Dose: once daily for five days.

Externally, the application of *Arnica, Ruta* and *Rhus* liniment will be very beneficial.

9.   Canker.   This is a chronic hypertrophy of the horn-producing tissues of the foot, especially of the hind-limb. Infection by necrotic bacilli takes place in the horn which has been softened by the animal standing for long periods in urine-soaked bedding or mud. The disease frequently runs a long course before signs appear.

SYMPTOMS

Lameness is evident. There is a specific odour associated with the condition and inspection of the foot reveals a ragged appearance of the frog, the tissue of which is easily removed, showing a cheese-like deposit underneath. The lesions are necrotic, slow to heal and bleed easily.

TREATMENT

Natrum muriaticum 200c This will help prevent extension of necrosis and hasten healing. Dose: once daily for one week.

Silicea 200c Useful in helping to harden the horn of the foot. Dose: once daily for five days.

Externally, after removal of dead tissue, the cavities should be packed with cotton-wool soaked in *Calendula* and *Arnica* lotions.

XXVI Affections of Fore and Hind Limbs

1. **Windgalls.**   This is a distension of a joint capsule, tendon-sheath or bursa with synovial fluid. The fetlock joint capsule is the one usually affected and swellings may be seen above and at the front of the seasmoid bones. When they affect the tendons, they occur between the suspensory ligaments and the flexor tendons.

SYMPTOMS
The swellings are usually tense because of the amount of synovial fluid in them but lameness is absent.

TREATMENT
Apis 30c   Will control the amount of synovial fluid and hasten its absorption. Dose: hourly for four doses.
Kili bichromicum 30c   Will help prevent the expression of synovial fluid through the skin. Dose: once daily for five days.
Externally, an application of *Arnica* and *Rhus* tox. liniments will be of great help in the healing process.

2. **Gravel.**   This is a term used to denote an infection which invades the sensitive structures through a crack in the white line. The lack of a drainage point permits the infection to reach the heel area where drainage may take place.

SYMPTOMS
Lameness varies according to the severity of the infection and the location of the original injury. Black spots appear on the white line and may penetrate to the laminae. Penetration of one or other of the black spots usually yields pus. Heel drainage occurs through time at the coronary band.

TREATMENT

Hepar sulphuris 200c　Will prevent suppuration if given early. Dose: once daily for four days.

Silicea 200c　Pyogenic infection will often yield to this remedy, which will also aid healing of necrotic tissue. Dose: once daily for five days.

Calarea fluorica 30c　Will promote hardening and granulation of tissue. Dose: once a week for four weeks.

Externally, any opening of black spots should be bathed with *calendula* lotion.

3. Thrush.　This is a degenerative condition of the frog and is accompanied by the presence of black necrotic material in the grooves. Prolonged involvement may cause spread to the horn and sensitive laminae. Lack of frog pressure may contribute to the condition along with unhygienic stabling, allowing entrance of the necrosis bacilus.

SYMPTOMS

Early signs include an increase of moisture on the frog and a black discharge from the grooves. The discharge has the characteristic odour of necrotic horn. The grooves of the frog become deeper than usual and the structure itself may be destroyed.

TREATMENT

Kreosotum 200c　Associated with constitutional upsets along with thrush, e.g. discharge from nose, offensive urine, etc. Dose: once daily for five days.

Silicea 200c　Will help healing necrotic tissue and promote healthy granulation. Dose: once daily for five days.

Kali bichromicum 30c　Discharge of offensive material. Dose: night and morning for seven days.

Externally, the grooves of the frog should be dressed early with plugs of cotton wool soaked in a lotion of *Calendula, Kali bich.* and *Arnica.*

4. Sandcrack.　Cracks in the wall of the hoof may commence from the coronary band or from the bearing surface of the wall, and may appear at the toe, quarter or heel. Lameness is not necessarily an accompaniement, but if infection gains entrance to the sensitive laminae through the crack it will result in suppuration and escape of purulent material through the crack or at the white line.

TREATMENT

Silicea 200c   Will help promote hardening and growth of new horn. Dose: once daily for five days.

Calcarea fluorica 30c   A good tissue remedy which will also promote horn growth. Dose: twice weekly for eight weeks.

Hepar sulphuris 1M   Infection in laminae. Dose: once daily for seven days.

Index

107; severe, 112
Epidermal cells, inflammation of, 76
Epidermis, 77
Epididymis, 109
Epistaxis—Nose Bleed, 21, 39, 44, 49, 50, 114, 128; treatment, 21-2
Epithelial cells, keratinisation of, 74
Equine Viral Arteritis, 118: symptoms, 119; treatment, 119
Equine Viral Rhinopheumonitis, 116-17, 119: Symptoms, 117; treatment, 117
Erysipeloid inflammation, 76
Erysipelatous inflammation, 76
Erythema, 78
Erythematous lesion, 77
Erythrocytes, 65
Eustachian tube, blockage in, 16
Excitement, 12: great, 106; sexual, 124
Exophthalmos, 33
Exostoses, 133, 153, 154, 160; bony, 150
Expectoration, 28: greenish, 30; profuse, 48; scanty, 31
Eye: bloodshot involvement, 44; engorgement of veins, 12; marked increase in size of, 13; reddish brown appearance of, 12
Eyeball: contusion of, 7: symptoms, 7; treatment, 7; in constant motion, 14; open wounds of, 7; treatment, 7-8; reduced tension in, 13
Eyelids: agglutination of, 12; closure of, 9, 19; heaviness of, 13; red, 13; swollen, 10, 22

Facial sinuses, pus in, 24: symptoms, 24; treatment, 24
Faeces: evil-smelling, 125; mucus and bright-red blood in, 124, 125; pale, 137
Faintness, 42
Febrile involvement, 29, 45, 69, 90, 119
Feet(oo): swelling of, 163; tenderness of, 116
Fever, 17, 18, 21, 99, 115, 119, 123, 125
Fibrosis, 156
Fibrous enlargements, 150
Fibular-tarsal bones, enlargement

of, 166
Fissuring, 80
Fistula, 4: symptoms, 4; treatment, 4-5
Fistulous involvement, 130
Flatulence, 35, 54, 57, 62, 85
Flatus, 17, 59, 60, 61: excessive, 63, 140; frequent passing of, 54; rumbling of, 61; very offensive, 54
Flexion, 163, 165: mild, 164; spasmodic, 164
Fluid, excess of, 97
Foci, suppurative, 82

Gait, 95: abduction, 34; faltering, 143; stiffness of, 145; tremulous or tottering, 51, 141
Gastric respiratory upset, symptoms of, 74
Gastritis, catarrhal, 56, 62
Genital organs: involvement of external, 116; ulceration of external, 121
Genital Tract Infection of Mares, 101: symptoms, 101; treatment, 101-2
Glomerulo-nephritis, 65: symptoms, 65; treatment, 65-6; acute, 65; chronic, 65
Gonitis, 163-4: symptoms, 164; treatment, 164
Grass Sickness, 138: symptoms, 138; treatment, 138-9: acute, 138; chronic, 138; sub-acute, 138
Gravel, 168: symptoms, 168-9; treatment, 169
Guttural pouch: pus in, 15, 99: symptoms, 15; treatment, 15; tympanitis of, 16: symptoms, 16; treatment, 16

Haematemesis, 39
Haematuria, 65, 66, 68: symptoms, 68; treatment, 68-9
Haemolysis, intravascular, 126
Haemolytic Anaemia of New Born Foals, 126: symptoms, 126; treatment, 127
Haemopoiesis, 123
Haemoptysis, 40
Haemorrhage(s), 5, 7, 8, 39, 89, 119, 132, 150-1: treatment,

Polymyositis, 92
Polyuria, 39, 66, 67, 68
Portal circulation, disturbance of, 63
Post-abortion discharges, 108
Prostration, 34, 57, 108
Pruritis, 3, 48, 78, 80: intense, 128; severe, 4, 77
Puerperal fever, 87
Puerperal involvement, 102
Pulmonary congestion, 26, 29, 30, 119: symptoms, 27; treatment, 27
Pulse: frequent rate, 30; decrease in rate, 30, 54; full, 12, 21, 25, 26, 29, 31, 32, 37, 46, 53, 55, 61, 65, 90, 99, 146, 159; hard, 34, 55, 145; irregular, 32, 33, 35, 36, 38, 44, 144; jugular, 37, 126; low tension, 33, 35; quickened, 25; rapid, 2, 8, 29, 33, 35, 45, 57, 87, 102, 125, 139, 141, 144, 158; slow, 33, 34, 38, 52, 70; small, 32; soft, 52; strong, 27; tense, 32; throbbing, 18; tremulous, 32, 35; weak, 33, 34, 38, 40, 41, 44, 58, 89, 125; wiry, 34, 145
Pupils: and contractions, 18; dilated, 21, 31, 45, 53, 55, 57, 61, 65, 90, 99, 146
Purpura haemorrhagica, 127, 128: symptoms, 127; treatment, 127-8
Purulent discharge, 3, 8, 12, 15, 22, 23, 24, 25, 90, 129, 159, 170
Purulent involvement, 8, 102
Pus, 10, 24, 157: creamy, 3, 90, 104; foul-smelling, 4; greenish, 2, 3, 4, 104; greyish, 5; p. in Guttural Pouch, 15: symptoms, 15; treatment, 15-16
Pyelonephritis, 71: symptoms, 71; treatment, 71-2; secondary, 72
Pyogenic infections, 47, 169
Pyogenic involvement, 75, 80, 110
Pyramidal Disease, 156: symptoms, 156; treatment, 156-7
Pyaemia, 117

Quittor, 157: symptoms, 157, treatment, 157

Radial Paralysis, 148: symptoms, 148; treatment, 148

Ranula, 51: symptoms, 51; treatment, 51; fluid in, 51
Rectal prolapse, 57
Rectum: bleeding from, 57; prolapse of, 60
Rectus femoris, 163
Recumbency, 96, 99, 106, 132, 134, 141, 145
Redness, 1
Resentment, 34, 64; of pressure, 118
Respiration: abdominal, 34; difficult, 144; increased, 65, 145; laboured, 61, 126; quickened, 25, 53, 58, 69, 70, 141, 158; rapid, 8; rattling sounds, 26; shallow, 2, 87; short, 61
Respiratory distress, 27, 33, 35, 40, 75; symptoms of, 74
Respiratory symptoms, 48, 78; prominence of, 33
Respiratory tract: affection of mucous membrane of, 28; catarrhal condition of, 24; infection of, 117, 118
Restlessness, 34, 54, 57, 58, 59, 60, 65, 74, 88, 103, 108, 111, 112, 117, 119, 138, 139, 145, 146
Retained placenta, 89
Retinitis, 11, 13
Rhinopneumonia, vaccination against, 126
Rickets, 95
Ringbone—Phalangeal Exostoses, 155: symptoms, 156; treatment, 156; articular, 155-6; High, 155, 156; Low, 155; periarticular, 156
Ringworm, 82: symptoms, 82; treatment, 82

Sacral region: pain over, 162; tenderness over, 145, 146
Saliva(tion), 8, 15, 25, 29, 47, 52, 54, 58, 88, 92, 100, 112, 132: accumulation of frothy, 30; no, 50; profuse, 50, 51; white, 51
Salmonella abortus-equi, 96
Salt metabolism, deficient, 42
Salt retention, 66
Sandcrack, 169-70; treatment, 170
Scalds, 5-6; treatment, 6
Scrotum, swelling of, 124